MW00561430

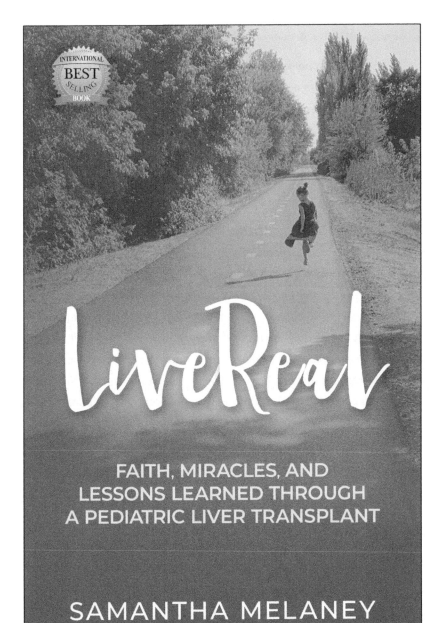

LiveReal

FAITH, MIRACLES, AND LESSONS LEARNED THROUGH A PEDIATRIC LIVER TRANSPLANT

SAMANTHA MELANEY

PRAISE FOR LIVEREAL

"This is a poignant description from the heart about the experience of an amazing family in loving and caring for a child who needs a liver transplant. I feel so privileged to be part of this journey as her 'liver doctor.'"

— **Linda Book MD**, Professor of Pediatrics University of Utah, Director Pediatric Liver Disease and Transplant Primary Children's Medical Center.

"I was honored to meet Samantha Melaney and her sweet family when I was their wish granter at Make-A-Wish Utah. I knew a little about their diagnosis at the time but now reading their story, Samantha fully brings you into her family's journey through liver transplant in an incredibly thoughtful and inspiring way. As scary as the reality is of having a sick child what's amazing is her positive spin on things that makes you realize the incredible resilience, hope and strength that one's faith can provide. Truly an inspirational and heartfelt book."

— **Tracy Silva,** Wish Granter,
Make-A-Wish Utah

"Samantha Melaney has written an intimate, heartfelt book bringing the world of pediatric liver transplant to life. From emotional moments of uncertainty, fear and doubt, Samantha demonstrates courage and perseverance. Her strength brings hope to us all."

— **Barbara Wilson**, LCSW,
Liver Transplant Social Worker,
Primary Children's Hospital

"Law school final exams require weeks of preparation and intensive study. Imagine studying for that exam while waiting to hear whether your hospitalized baby girl needs a liver transplant. Zachary Melaney found a way to balance the two, and he still took the time to send thank you notes to his professors for accommodating his family emergency. I can't imagine anyone else handling such a trying time with such strength and integrity."

— **Jessica M. Kiser,** Associate Professor,
Gonzaga University School of Law

"I watched Zach and Samantha parent their children during the most difficult of times. As I read the book, I realized they went through more adversity than I originally thought. Zach and Samantha's diligence and champion parenting along with medical ingenuity saved Kendyl's life and their journey is an example to all about navigating difficult times in life."

— **Cari Fullerton**, Executive VP, Chief Credit Officer
Bank of Utah

"I was immediately DRAWN in this powerful story, as if I was a close family member experiencing this along with the family. As a mother myself, I couldn't imagine going through these moments with my daughter. Samantha takes us on the journey with her through Live Real, it is wrenching and full of beauty at the same time. Her message "remember to celebrate others' victories as you wait for your own" is powerful and is now a quote in my phone! Thank you Samantha."

— **Danielle Amos**, Success Mindset Coach, CEO,
www.danielleamos.co

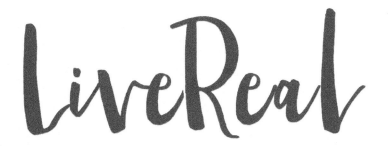

LiveReal

Faith, Miracles, and Lessons Learned Through a Pediatric Liver Transplant

Samantha Melaney

GLOBAL WELLNESS MEDIA
STRATEGIC EDGE INNOVATIONS PUBLISHING
LOS ANGELES, TORONTO, MONTREAL

For permission requests, send an email to book@samanthamelaney.com

First Edition. Published by:
Global Wellness Media
Strategic Edge Innovations Publishing
340 S Lemon Ave #2027
Walnut, California 91789-2706
(866) 467-9090
StrategicEdgeInnovations.com

Editors: Lisa Jones, Eric. D. Groleau
Book Design: Global Wellness Media
Cover Design: Eric D. Groleau

LiveReal / Samantha Melaney. -- 1st ed.
ISBN: 978-1-7363047-9-2 (Kindle)
ISBN: 978-1-957343-92-1 (Paperback)

DISCLAIMER

The information contained herein is not intended to be a substitute for professional evaluation and therapy with a health professional. If you are experiencing any health issues, you need to seek professional help.

This book is based on the author's personal experience and other real-life examples. To protect privacy, some names or details may have been modified.

DEDICATION

This book is dedicated to my strong daughters, Alyx and Kendyl.

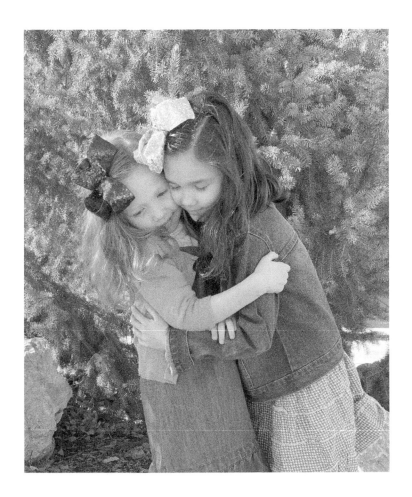

TABLE OF CONTENTS

FOREWORD

I'll never forget the day I was walking to the hospital to see Kendyl again. It was one of the most difficult weeks of my life. I had traveled back to Spokane for her first major surgery. I had gone by myself, and due to complicated circumstances, I was staying at a hotel somewhat close to the hospital so that I could walk back and forth. At the end of each long day, I would go to my room exhausted and worried, but my racing thoughts about "why ... how ... and what if..." wouldn't let me sleep.

It had snowed heavily, and the cold, slushy roads seemed to fit the situation. My heart was heavy, and the future seemed as dreary as the weather. But that day, as I was walking to the hospital trying not to slip on the wet roads, this distinct thought came to my mind: *"Kendyl is a fighter. She's not going to give up."*

This is a story about our little girl, Kendyl Rose, who has proven over the past years that the thought that came to my mind was not just wishful thinking, but a clear impression. Unfortunately, she has had more than enough opportunities to show her fighting spirit. This story also shows that the impression was not just about Kendyl, but about her mom, dad, sister, and her entire family.

Kendyl received a feeding tube when she was four months old. It was difficult to see her with a tube going down her nose and tape on her beautiful little face, but we knew it was needed. One day, when Kendyl was home, she pulled her feeding tube out. We had no idea what we were going to do! Samantha called the home health nurse and explained the situation. She was kind enough to come to the house and put the tube back in. We expressed our appreciation for her assistance and asked if we could call her next time Kendyl would pull it out. I don't recall her exact words, but she said something about how Samantha would need to do it next time. I couldn't believe it! "How can you expect a young mother to do that?", I thought. The next four years showed me that Sam is also a fighter, she doesn't give up, and that her love for her daughter would help her do things I hoped my daughter would never have to do. I'll always be grateful for her consistent, diligent, loving efforts to give her daughter the best care possible.

Zach was in his last year of law school when Kendyl was born and later diagnosed. I was so impressed at how he continued to do his best to keep up with his studies while so much was going on in his family's life. His positive attitude is a gift, but at times, I would get frustrated when he didn't seem to understand the seriousness of the situation. However, my frustration turned to gratitude. We all needed his optimistic, hopeful outlook. Zach is a fighter, and he never gave up on Kendyl, his schooling, or on his responsibility as a husband and a father.

Alyx, our beautiful, funny, chatty, constantly singing entertainer. Her life has been altered due to her little sister's medical condition, but God knew Kendyl needed Alyx. Our whole family needed Alyx! Her singing and dancing lightened our mood. Watching her introduce herself to complete strangers in the hospital brought us much needed laughs after long, discouraging days. A and K were meant to be together, even though they spent much time apart in their early years. Alyx has always been the protective, loving big sister. She's a fighter, and with every hospital stay, she never gave up hoping that her little sister would "be home soon."

The list of fighters, those who never gave up on Kendyl during her entire journey, is long. It also includes her grandparents, aunts, uncles, and cousins. All the amazing medical professionals who cared for her through every challenge and cheered after every victory. Her donor and their family, who chose to turn their tragedy into a life-saving gift. Her neighbors and friends who gave of their means, time, support, and love. And although God may have seemed silent in some of our darkest moments, we know He was there fighting for us and with us from the very beginning of the journey. He never gave up on our family.

I had a front-row seat to this story. For a while, it seemed like the heaviness of our situation would never end, and there were times I really thought my heart was going to break. I will always wish that Kendyl had been born with a healthy liver. She will deal with the challenges of living with a liver transplant for the rest of her life. However, her story and our experiences have taught me a few things: Angels are among us, and they roam the halls of homes and hospitals. Watching your children learn how strong they really are is one of the hardest and most rewarding experiences a parent can have. Miracles still happen every day.

Kendyl's scars will always be a visible reminder of her fight to live and the miracles we witnessed. Unlike her scars, the changes her journey made in me are not visible but will be a part of me forever. They will never fade, and I will always be so grateful for them. Thank you Kendyl for being such a fighter, and for never giving up. Grandma loves you to pieces!

Lisa Jones

INTRODUCTION

This book is meant to provide hope and support to parents who might be going through similar experiences, but it is also written to inspire people dealing with challenging moments.

While relating our story, it also highlights powerful lessons that we have drawn along with strengths that we discovered along the way. What initially started as a project to record our journey for our daughters, soon expanded into this book, which I hope, will provide courage and faith to many families.

Samantha Melaney

PREFACE

Late in the summer of 2013, I remember saying out loud several times, "We won't have a baby until we move back." This was my mindset when we moved from West Haven, Utah to Spokane, Washington for Zach to attend school at Gonzaga University, pursuing a JD/MBA dual degree. I felt strongly about this decision for several reasons, such as having a difficult pregnancy and severe post-partum depression with my first baby. It also made sense financially to wait until we were done with school.

However, in the fall of 2014, I began to have strong feelings that it was time for us to grow our family. It is a good thing that I didn't know what was coming and how much of a journey we were starting by simply having another baby, while living away from family. Despite all we have been through, I can honestly say I would do it again and it was all worth it.

Chapter 1

LiveReal

2015

January 31, 2015

I took a pregnancy test and learned I was pregnant when I saw the two lines on the stick. I was excited to grow our family and be able to give Alyx a sibling. The excitement carried me for the following nine hard months. I'm not someone who likes to be pregnant. If you are one of those people, I'm not sure we can be friends. Seriously, though.

Just like my first pregnancy, I threw up basically the whole time. (I think there might have been a stretch of about six weeks where I didn't, but that was about it.) I felt so sick, tired, and uncomfortable. When I was pregnant with my first, it was OK because Zach could take care of himself. This second one was a lot harder because I had a two-year-old in tow. I'm still not quite sure how I kept her alive during a second pregnancy, while Zach was in school.

May 18, 2015

My prediction of having a girl was confirmed and we were so excited. It was fun to have Zach there with me and hearing that everything looked good with our little one. As soon as she told us it was a girl, I pictured having all things pink, Barbies, dance recitals, drama, and all the girly stuff. I was so excited for Alyx to have a sister.

That night we decorated a big box that said, "Boy or Girl" and had balloons in it for Alyx to unbox. We called both sides of our families on FaceTime video and they all screamed with excitement when they saw the four pink balloons come out of the box. It was a fun day, and we immediately began talking about names and envisioning our future as a family of four with two little girls.

September 25, 2015

It was a LONG nine months, but we made it. I took pictures of my belly and our last picture as a family of three before going to the hospital. Having a scheduled C-section takes the unknown and some of the excitement out. Being the planner that I like to be, it probably worked out best this way.

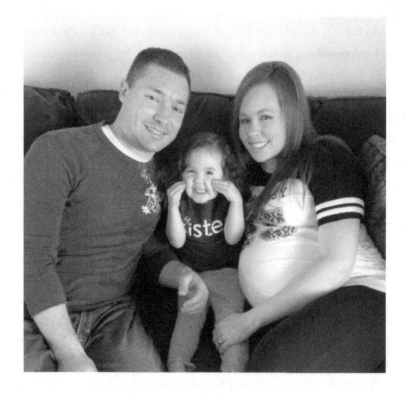

Both of our parents came to Washington from Utah to meet their new granddaughter. We arrived early and as they prepped me for delivery. I couldn't wait to meet my new little girl and watch my oldest become a big sister.

Our beautiful Kendyl Rose Melaney was born, and she was the sweetest little thing! It was such a wonderful and happy day as all went well during delivery. It was wonderful to have our family there with us. We all took turns holding Kendyl and celebrating this precious girl and loving on her dark full head of hair. It melted my heart to watch Alyx meet her. She held her and said, "Hi, I'm your big sister." The hospital was one block away from our home, so Zach stayed with me most of the time. Each night he would go home to get Alyx to bed and then come back to see me while our parents stayed with her.

September 27, 2015

The stay in the hospital was uneventful. We returned home and started our journey as a family of four. A few days later our family members went home except my mom who stayed with us to help for a few weeks.

Not many people know this, but Kendyl didn't pass her hearing test before we left the hospital, so she had to be tested a few days after we were discharged. The doctor was pretty sure that happened because I had a C-section (which I guess is common) but she needed another test to be sure. I wasn't too worried about her hearing because I had noticed that she would react to loud noises and other things around her, but I still kept saying to myself, "What if something was wrong?" I kept repeating that in my head for days leading up to the appointment. I was relieved when she passed the hearing test, but I never seemed to snap out the feeling of "What if something was wrong with my baby?"

I believe God knows us individually and knows what we need. To me, this was a tender mercy that prepared me a little for something that was wrong with my sweet little baby, before we knew it.

Current challenges prepare us for future ones.

October 2015

My mom had planned to stay four weeks when Kendyl was born. The first three weeks of her life were an absolute bliss. It didn't even feel real. I had tried to prepare myself for sleepless nights and being tired but that wasn't the case. She slept a lot, she didn't cry much, and was the best little snuggler. She had a sweet and loving spirit about her. This is something that is still true today. She gives the BEST hugs ever.

I felt I was rocking this newborn life. I had this 2-kids thing down. It was about this moment when I started to feel it was time for my mom to go back home. Not in a bad way, but I felt like she needed to get back to her life in Utah and I believed I had everything under control.

At the fourth week of Kendyl's life, things began to change. She started to spit up everywhere and all the time. She would throw up constantly and she became super fussy and irritable. Kendyl seemed to change overnight, and I didn't feel like she was the same baby. I would nurse her at night, about 8 p.m. to put her to sleep, and then by 11 p.m. I would still be rocking her and trying to get her to sleep. I would nurse her again and usually get her down for the night between midnight and 2 a.m. This started to happen every day. As a new mom, it became exhausting quickly and I wondered what happened to my easy baby.

I remember when my mom told me how long she would stay, I thought that seemed like a long time for her to be away from home and her own responsibilities, but I couldn't get her to change her mind. That fourth week, when I thought that I was doing fine but Kendyl started becoming fussy, I knew that my mom had been right. I can't imagine how I would've handled things at that point without her help.

October 2015

Before my mom left, she spent hours researching natural and other remedies to help Kendyl and her symptoms. She ordered many things on Amazon for us to try and we went to Babies "R" US to look at potential remedies. While being in the store, I remember my mom talking to my dad on the phone and telling him that we thought Kendyl might have some reflux or something else, while describing how fussy she was and how often she threw up. We even bought a mamaRoo swing that day in hopes that the motion would soothe her.

I recall thinking that I had been so dumb that day to think I had everything under control and realized just how much I needed my mom. As my dad mentioned on the phone that he was excited for my mom to come back, I felt like saying, "No. She can't come back. I need her here. I have no idea what I'm doing." My mom tried to do everything she could to help before leaving. We had ordered so many things to try, so she believed something would help and went home as scheduled. It was a sad day for all of us, but especially for Alyx and I since it was fun to have her there with us. She helped so much, which was welcomed as Zach was studying at school. I said goodbye and held on to the excitement that she would be back soon, when Kendyl would be blessed in church.

Kendyl was still throwing up, so I decided to take her to the pediatrician. I had noticed that her diapers didn't look normal. There wasn't much color to them, and it seemed foamy. I asked the pediatrician about it; while she never saw one of her diapers, she reassured me it was OK. I was happy to know that Kendyl had reflux, and she was gaining weight. I was relieved to know that it wasn't something serious.

I learned that if you are worried about something, it never hurts to look deeper into it, especially with little ones. I'm grateful that I took her in to the doctor that day. The visit helped me to feel more at peace about why she was throwing up so much. She seemed to improve over the next few weeks, and I felt reassured that the medicine she was taking was what she needed. I was so grateful she was doing better.

November 26, 2015

It was the first year both Zach and I had Thanksgiving without our families. I spent most of the day cooking, while Zach held Kendyl and played with Alyx. It was a small celebration, but it was also a great day. It was fun for me to have a little mom break and to cook. It felt good to provide my little family with a nice meal. I was happy that Kendyl was doing better and felt so much gratitude for all my blessings, especially my husband and two little girls.

December 1, 2015

I was feeling proud that with two kids, and one being a new baby, I was all ready for Christmas. In mid-November I had this strong feeling to be ready early. At the time, it made sense to me because we were planning to go back home for Christmas and surprise both of our families. I felt that it would be a good idea to be ready early and figure out what gifts were going to Utah and which ones were staying, etc.

It felt good to know I was prepared, and we even bought our first little Christmas tree that was up before our parents arrived in early December. Having the Christmas tree up for their visit helped me feel more confident that we could convince them that we were staying in Spokane for Christmas, even though the plan was to fly to Utah and surprise them.

You never know the reason for a prompting or a feeling. Sometimes, you might think you know why you have the thoughts and feelings, yet it could be a totally different reason.

Listen to your feelings, whether you
know why you have them or not.

December 4, 2015

I had heard a few friends talk about this holiday light show in Coeur d'Alene, Idaho, that happens only at Christmas time. It was about 40 minutes from our home so I thought it would be a fun way to kick off the Christmas season. My in-laws were coming up a few days before Kendyl's blessing, so we decided this would be a fun activity for all of us.

The show starts as you get on a boat and ride along the lake, looking at the beautiful Christmas lights leading up to the North Pole. As you arrive, you see Santa from a distance, and he mentions all the children's names on the nice list. Kendyl was in a carrier on my chest; it was fun to snuggle her while being out and about and watching Alyx enjoy it.

I am grateful for this memory as it ended up being the only Christmas activity we did the whole season.

If you have an opportunity to make a memory, don't miss out. You might never have another chance.

December 6, 2015

One of the happiest days of my entire life was Kendyl's blessing day. It was fun to have both my parents and my in-laws in town for the occasion. I remember that morning so well. I was curling my hair when my father-in-law came upstairs and said, "I need you to come downstairs so that I can give you your Christmas present." I'll admit, I was a little bugged and wondered why I couldn't finish my hair first, but we all went downstairs. As we waited, I heard footsteps. Then more footsteps. Next thing I knew Zach's sister was coming down the stairs, then his other sister. I couldn't believe it! Then his brother, his other brother, etc. until all six of Zach's siblings were standing in their church clothes in our basement. They came all the way from Utah for the occasion. I still remember looking at them with my jaw WIDE open. It felt like a dream. I kept pinching myself to see if this was real.

9

While I hurried to finish getting ready, I didn't care about my hair as much. As I got in the car, with our family following us to our church, I looked around and just took in the moment. It was a feeling of happiness and gratitude that is still hard to describe. I remember that drive to church, looking at the beautiful place that we lived, looking at my cute husband, my adorable girls, and seeing all of our family following us for this special day. I kept thinking how blessed I was to be with my loving family, Zach was in his last year of JD/MBA school, and I felt so much happiness and pure joy. Life was so good and our future looked bright. What could possibly go wrong?

It was a beautiful day. Zach gave a wonderful blessing, and it was great to have not only both of our fathers, but also four uncles that we didn't expect to be there in the circle. It was also nice to not worry about Kendyl throwing up. She looked beautiful in her dress, and it was special that it was the same dress Alyx wore for her baby blessing too. We enjoyed taking pictures of everyone there. After church, we came home and made breakfast food for lunch. It is a Melaney family tradition to have breakfast food for lunch on the first Sunday of the month, and it was great to be carrying on the tradition in our home in Spokane. After lunch, the siblings went and toured the law school to see where Zach spent most of his days. It was fun for them to see where their little brother was studying. We had a wonderful evening and a memory I hope to never forget. This was a perfect blessing, which helped strengthen us for the storm that was coming.

I was sad when it was time for them to leave. It was a very short trip. They flew from Utah to Washington in the morning and headed back that same night. I still remember my pregnant sister-in-law's swollen feet and how bad I felt for her. We have all said what a great memory it was for all of us. The siblings enjoyed flying together and it was fun for Zach and I to have them with us. Many said that the moment they first held Kendyl, they could feel that she was special. Her blessing day truly was one of the happiest days of my life.

I'm still shocked that this big surprise of the siblings coming was not spoiled. As we talked about it later, they said it was so hard not to mention anything when we would do a FaceTime call. Definitely one of the biggest surprises of my life. Looking back, there were a few minor clues. When we bought the food for Sunday, I couldn't figure out why my father-in-law was encouraging us to get more food. Even with his few comments, I had no suspicion of the surprise that was coming. It's always fun to look back at the signs that you missed or didn't notice at the time. I'm grateful that I was oblivious. It was perfect.

December 7, 2015

The day after Kendyl's blessing, both my in-laws and my dad left to head home while my mom stayed with us for the rest of the week. We had decided to do something fun that morning, before taking my dad to the airport. However, Kendyl started throwing up a lot and I was nervous to take her anywhere, so we ended up just staying home. I felt bad that we didn't do anything enjoyable before my dad left. I also started to wonder again if something was wrong. I thought the medicine was what she needed, but it now felt like we were back to where we had started. We had an appointment later that week and I was anxious to see what the doctor would say this time.

There are blessings and tender moments all around us, but we must notice them. It is easy to see things as coincidences and not think too much of those situations, but if you take a chance to notice, you might realize how truly blessed you are. As I look back, having that medicine work for a short amount of time was an absolute tender mercy for me. I remember vividly being so grateful and not worried about Kendyl throwing up on her blessing day. I know it is a silly thing, but it meant a lot to me. I didn't have to stress about it that day and truly feel that I enjoyed that day to the fullest. It was just one day later, when suddenly, the medicine didn't seem to work anymore. I'm not sure why it worked for a couple of weeks because we would realize later that reflux was not the problem. Yet, I am truly grateful for her blessing day and the days before, when the medicine seemed to work. I truly know in my heart that it was a blessing and a tender mercy.

December 11, 2015

My mom was once again heading home. She took a darling video of Kendyl, babbling in her bouncer that morning, as she kept talking back to her. It was a precious video. When we arrived at the airport, my mom gave Kendyl a kiss and told her that she loved her. My mom gave all the love she could before leaving. She had this feeling that, "no matter what happens, families are eternal, and we will all be together forever someday."

Just as every other time my mom had come to visit, I cried as we said goodbye. But this time, I was feeling proud of myself that I was able to cry and act as though I wasn't coming home for Christmas. I then went straight to the pediatrician's office for Kendyl's appointment. I remember waiting in the waiting room longer than anticipated. When we finally got to the room, I was feeling overwhelmed dealing with both girls by myself. As we waited in the room for the doctor, she threw up three times. When her doctor finally came in, she looked her over and asked me, "Does she look yellow to you?" I replied with, "Um... I don't know." I was a little annoyed and thought how would I know? I stare at her every day.

Her weight was hardly up at all from our last visit, when I was told she had reflux. I had tried to tell myself that the lack of weight gain was because of her throwing up. The doctor decided to get some blood work and at this moment, the feeling in the room changed. I didn't know what, but I knew something was wrong with my baby. The blood draw was difficult as both girls were there with me, and I had the sinking feeling of knowing, before the blood was even taken, that those results were going to show something wrong and unsettling. The doctor said that she would be in touch. I had no idea what to think, but I could feel in my heart that something was obviously wrong.

As we left the pediatrician's office, tears streamed down my face and worry filled my mind. Even though Zach was at school, I called him immediately. I told him something was wrong with Kendyl and told him about the visit. Being the loving husband that he is, he said, "I'm sure everything will be OK, but do you want to pick me up from school now?" Yes, I said as I drove straight to the law school. It was a Friday but still much earlier than he would normally leave school. By the time I picked him up, he had done some of his own research on Google and once again, lovingly reassured me that all would be well. I wasn't very convinced. As soon as I saw him come out of the school, I jumped out of the car and let him drive home because I was too upset. I went home and didn't know what to do. I couldn't seem to focus on anything. I couldn't call my mom (as I would usually do in these situations) because she was on a plane heading home. I kept pacing the floor, asking out loud, "What is wrong with my baby? Why would we not know until now?"

Finally, the pediatrician called and told me the results of the blood work. Kendyl's bilirubin was high (7.5), so she needed to be seen by a physician. In my mind, I thought oh, OK, I'll bring her on Monday … and then I heard her say, "I have set up a room at Sacred Heart Hospital. Take her there immediately." Her final words rang in my mind. "Unfortunately, when I usually see these things, it is something serious."

I hung up the phone and told Zach what she had said. I had never been to that hospital before in my life (as Kendyl was born in a different hospital) and I didn't want to go alone. I didn't want to call someone on late notice, and I wanted Zach there with me. At that moment, I wished more than anything that we weren't 700 miles away from family. I didn't have much info yet and didn't want to talk to anyone. We drove as a family to the hospital. Zach dropped Kendyl and me at the door and then went to park with Alyx. I walked in and they started asking questions, but I could tell that they were indeed ready for us. They got us settled in a room and a few minutes later, Zach and Alyx joined us.

It was the first time that night when I heard of a liver disease called Biliary Atresia. I couldn't understand it when they first said those words and it took days before I learned what the disease was, how to say it, and what it meant. Biliary Atresia is a life-threatening liver disease that blocks the ducts that carry bile from the liver to the gallbladder. As the bile gets backed up, it destroys the liver.

After about an hour or so, Alyx started to get restless and hungry, so Zach took her home for dinner and put her to bed. I felt so incredibly alone in this new hospital as I wondered what the future would hold. (I could have never imagined what was ahead of us.)

I had waited until then to send something to my mom because I didn't want to worry her, but I knew I'd better tell her now. I sent her a text that said something like, "Kendyl's appointment didn't go well, and we have been admitted to the hospital, but everything is OK" hoping she wouldn't worry.

I can't imagine how my mom felt when she read my text. She later told me she was waiting at the luggage carousel when she received my message. She told me her initial reaction was to grab her luggage and head back to the terminal so she could fly back to Spokane.

She called me immediately to talk. I didn't have much information, but I told her what happened after she left. As a mother, I can't imagine how she felt. She offered to fly back but I told her not to. It was best to see what was wrong first and go from there.

They did an ultrasound at around 11 p.m. that night. I was exhausted. It had been an emotional day and I felt so alone. I knew Zach was where he needed to be (with Alyx) but I wished so badly for him to be here with me. I was told that I would know the results of the tests the next day.

That night was LONG! We had to share a hospital room with a stranger with a fussy baby, and that mother wasn't very understanding. It was so upsetting. It was a long night with more tears than sleep.

There are moments that you never forget. No matter how hard you try, you can't. For me, one of those moments was that day at the

14

doctor's office and the dreaded phone call that followed. For my mom, I know that one of those moments was when that terrible text message came in.

Emotional impacts change us.

December 12, 2015

Zach came the next morning and the word started to get out. It wasn't long before a friend heard the news and came to the hospital to give Kendyl a blessing. It meant so much that he would come visit us on a busy Saturday. As he left, he shook our hands and slipped Zach $50 in cash. As we tried to tell him that we were OK, he said, "Life gets expensive in emergencies" and told us to keep it. This was such a kind act. Our friend probably doesn't remember this, but we do, and we always will. This visit, including a blessing for Kendyl and the donation, was a bright spot during a very dark time and taught me to follow through if I have an idea to help someone.

December 2015

The following days are a blur as Kendyl and I continued to stay at the hospital. We had meetings with doctors, blood draws, ultrasounds, and more. My mom flew back to Spokane a few days later and my in-laws also came back. It was fun to be together again so soon, but it was under heartbreaking circumstances. It was determined that Kendyl most likely had biliary atresia, but we wouldn't know for sure until they did a surgery called Kasai. The Kasai surgery removes the blocked bile ducts and gallbladder and replaces them with a segment of the small intestine. We knew it was major surgery and it was hard to imagine my baby, a week shy of three months old, would be going through this.

As we heard the possible diagnosis of biliary atresia, we began to Google it, which is never a good idea. One of the first things that came up as we searched were pictures of stool. As we looked at the pictures, it was getting clear that Kendyl most likely had this horrible disease. Even Google confirmed it was horrible.

To this day, we believe that if we had thought to Google pictures of stool (but why would you want to do that?), we may have realized her diagnosis earlier. But we didn't. Sure, that might have helped us get the diagnosis sooner, which is recommended, but I truly feel it was good that we never thought to research it. I am glad that we didn't find it that way. Beware of Google! Especially during stressful times. You are often going to find the worst-case scenario and horror stories. A diagnosis is never easy but there are some happy endings.

As we prepared for surgery, we met with the surgeon, Dr. G. I was impressed after meeting with him and even more so after looking him up online and reading that he was an amazing surgeon. It was comforting to know Kendyl was going to be in good hands.

We met with him a few times. One day, he had a darling 4-year-old girl and her mom join us. While the daughter colored a picture for us, they explained that she had received the same diagnosis and had the same Kasai surgery that Kendyl would be having. The surgery had been successful for her, and I truly felt in my heart that it would be the same for our little girl. I also remember when they would go over the success rate of the surgery that the next plan, if this didn't work, would be a liver transplant. I didn't even consider or give it any thought. I was sure that it was going to be successful.

Life now seemed to make more sense. Both Zach and I were very hopeful that he would be accepted into a law school in Utah. However, God had other plans for us, and we ended up moving from Utah to Washington for him to attend school. Now that we had found this amazing surgeon, who was very well known for Kasai surgery, it all seemed to make sense why Zach was accepted here.

We decided that the surgery would be Thursday, December 17th, a week after our world had fallen apart. Kendyl had been in the hospital for a week already, but that day seemed to work out best with the surgeon's schedule and Zach's final exam of the semester was that morning.

I remember when we were deciding a date for the surgery. I wanted it done immediately, the very next day. We had been told that the surgery was more successful when the child was younger, before the liver gets too damaged. However, my family and the surgeon nicely reminded me that a couple of days wouldn't make that much of a difference and that we should do what was best for everyone's schedules. Although we were living our lives in complete survival mode, Zach's finals were important for our future too. Sometimes, you can't see the big picture when you are in the middle of something scary but loved ones around you can. Let them help you to see what you might be missing.

In stressful times, it is always helpful to
have people around you that can provide
other insights you might not see.

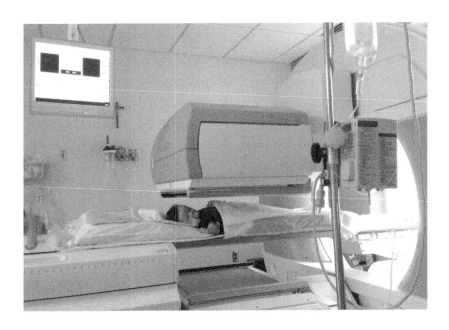

December 14, 2015

As we prepared for the Kasai surgery, Kendyl had something called a hepatobiliary iminodiacetic acid (or HIDA) scan. This is an imaging procedure used to diagnose problems of the liver, gallbladder, and bile ducts. This would gather information for the surgery. It is hard to forget the memory of seeing my tiny baby in this big tunnel, watching the screens showing her insides, and trying to read into the results.

December 16, 2015

One day before surgery, we were all feeling pretty nervous and anxious. While preparing for this, the GI doctor thought it would be helpful to meet a little boy and his mom who were in the hospital for a minor setback. He had had the same surgery when he was about Kendyl's age and was now doing well. He was a cutie and he looked to be a thriving and busy little boy.

However, he did have a little IV (intravenous) in his hand. Even if this was minor, it was something we weren't used to seeing. As the doctor was trying to help us feel better, it still felt overwhelming. I kept thinking, "OK, he is thriving, but he is still in the hospital."

The mom was very encouraging about the surgery. We still felt anxious, but it was comforting to meet others who knew what we were going through. When you first receive news of a diagnosis, it feels like you are all alone. We had never even heard of the disease, let alone knew someone with it. However, we began meeting many people who were familiar with the disease.

December 17, 2015

I didn't sleep much the night before. I got up feeling tired, emotional, and overwhelmed as I tried to somewhat get ready for the day. I couldn't believe that my baby was going in for a major surgery. My mom came to the hospital early (she was staying at a hotel near the hospital) and we gave Kendyl a bath. I wanted her to be all clean because I wasn't sure when I would be able to bathe her again after surgery. My mom took pictures of her bare belly, knowing that this was the last time her tummy would be scar-free. We didn't know then that her scars would later be a reminder of how tough she is, and how merciful God is. After getting her bathed, my mom gave me a little gift that was from another family member. I opened it to find a beautiful necklace that said, "Have Faith." I cried as I realized how much I needed that reminder on that day. Then my mom pulled out a necklace from under her shirt to show me that she had the same one. It was so thoughtful to not only give one to me, but to both of us. I will never forget that act of thoughtfulness and kindness and I still have the necklace today.

Zach wasn't there that morning as he was taking his last final. We were hoping that he would get to the hospital in time before they took her back for surgery. I was trying hard to keep it together as I looked at my beautiful baby girl, still not totally believing something was wrong with her. When I looked at her, it wasn't obvious that something was wrong, which made it harder. She was a little yellow, especially in her eyes, but I don't think that a stranger looking at my baby would have noticed.

They had us wait in a small waiting room. Me, Kendyl, my mom, my mother and father-in-law, and eventually Zach. We sat in that room passing a box of tissues back and forth as we cried, worried and silently prayed. I remember holding Kendyl and just crying. I didn't know it at the time, but my mom took a picture that says a thousand words. You can see the complete heartache and worry of a mother before they took her daughter to the operating room. I'm grateful that I have that picture from my mom as capturing the moment was the last thing I was thinking about.

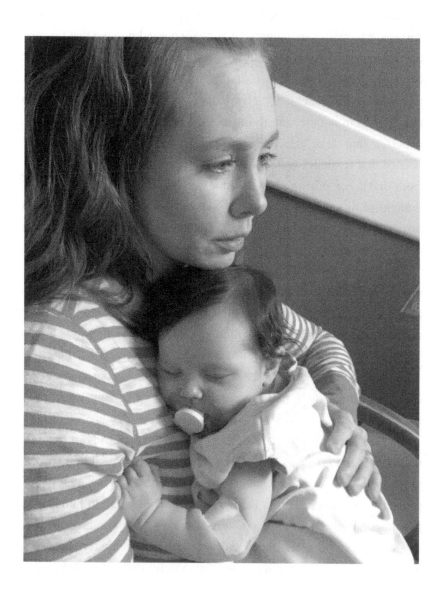

I will never forget placing my little baby into the arms of the doctors and wishing them good luck. It was an awful feeling as a mother. As a parent, you want to protect your kids and keep them safe. I felt in some way that I was letting my baby down.

The next hours were a blur until we finally were told we could see her. We couldn't wait to get back to her side but the first few minutes after seeing her broke my heart. They had tried to warn me. They told me there would be wires, etc. but when I looked at her, I cried and thought, "What did they do to my baby?" She had wires, markings, blood, drains, and it was so hard to witness. I felt immediately overwhelmed as I wondered how I would care for her or if I was strong enough to do so.

We had a postoperative discussion with the surgeon. He confirmed she did have biliary atresia, but there were a few other findings too. We learned that she had multiple spleens, which is known as polysplenia. We were told that she had at least four spleens (most people have one) and they were all intermingled. The surgeon also found that she had an artery that was out of place, but it was moved to where it should be. The findings from the surgery let us know that her condition was congenital, so there since birth. Not all cases of biliary atresia include other findings, like this, but it is common. During surgery they also removed her gallbladder, which had never worked properly. It was heartbreaking to hear the confirmed diagnosis.

> Even if you have warnings that something is coming, you never truly know what it is like until you are in that situation.

While I had prepped myself to see Kendyl like that and I thought I was ready. The doctors and nurses had tried to warn me, but I clearly wasn't. There was no way I would have been ready until being forced to be in that moment.

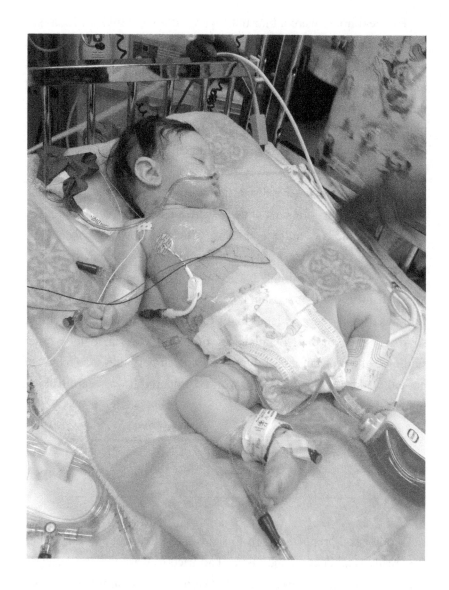

December 18, 2015

We were amazed to witness the love that was shown to Kendyl and our family during this time. I was touched by all the messages, texts, and phone calls we received. It felt like I couldn't keep up with everyone and with all the love that was expressed towards us. It truly meant so much to know we weren't alone at a time when life was so dark and heavy. Some of the support was from close friends but I was amazed that a lot was coming from people I had never met but just knew from social media. Shortly after the surgery, some friends from the neighborhood came to the hospital. We weren't expecting them, but it truly meant so much. One of them gave us a gift that was a darling sign that said, "Though she be little, she is fierce." I had never heard that phrase before, but I love it. It still hangs in Kendyl's room today.

People really do care. They truly are kind and thoughtful. I tried my best to post updates on social media during this time to keep friends and family members informed. I never expected the incredible amount of love that would be shown and felt, in so many ways, from family, friends, and strangers.

December 20, 2015

Kendyl was moved from the PICU (pediatric intensive care unit) to the regular floor. I was able to hold her for the first time since surgery. I was so nervous and worried that it would cause her pain. The nurses helped tremendously as they were able to move her with the wires. As I held her, I was amazed by her happy smile. She was a tiny baby, only three days post-surgery, yet she was smiling. It was a reminder of the strength she had and an example to always be happy.

From this day on, Kendyl has taught us this lesson over and over.

We can choose to be happy,
no matter our circumstances.

December 2015

I remember coming home one night while Zach was at the hospital with Kendyl. It was difficult to be home and remember what it was like before everything happened and reflect on what we had just been through. There was a stack of mail on our kitchen table and some packages. I started to go through the packages, and I realized that many of them were different remedies that my mom had ordered when she was here for the blessing, before we knew that something was wrong. I laughed thinking about the time and money we had spent on things we thought would solve Kendyl's issue. While I sat there laughing, a part of me wished that these remedies would have been what she needed.

Sometimes, you just need to laugh. Crying hurts my eyes and makes me much more tired than laughing.

The next few weeks were a blur. We were living the typical hospital life. I stayed at the hospital with Kendyl and Zach was at home with Alyx. We had amazing friends who watched Alyx, which allowed Zach to visit us. We will forever be grateful for all they did to help us in our time of need.

There were so many extreme feelings. Some were obvious, such as heartbreak and overwhelm, and others were feelings that most people probably wouldn't know, unless they were in similar situations, such as guilt. As an example, when I initially heard the news about my baby, I wondered if I had somehow caused this. Was it something I did during pregnancy? Perhaps it was the Nacho Cheese Doritos and Twizzlers licorice that I lived on for a month during pregnancy? (I was sure that was the case.) If you have never been in such a situation, these thoughts might sound absurd. But when you are going through something like this, you truly begin to wonder. I felt guilty that I might have caused this, and that I was responsible for everything Kendyl was going through. This was something that I had to work through and slowly let go as I was reassured over and over that the cause of biliary atresia is unknown.

As hard as it was to hear, everything made sense once we knew the diagnosis. It helped us realize why she was an angel for the first three weeks of life, when her liver wasn't yet blocked with bile, and why she got fussy and irritable shortly after. This also explains why her weight looked great at both her three-day-old and two-month-old appointments, but then later her weight increase stopped. Bile helps with the digestion of food, including the fats we consume. Without bile, the fats went right through Kendyl's system, so she wasn't getting the fats she needed to gain weight. As I learned more about this disease that had turned our lives upside down, I realized how much the liver truly does for our body. I don't think I had ever once thought about my liver before this diagnosis. I had always taken it for granted.

One of the many nights in the hospital, as I was trying to fall asleep, I realized how lucky we were that the pediatrician had noticed that something was wrong. I loved that pediatrician! Although I still wish the diagnosis could have been caught earlier, it was still found promptly. I felt grateful for this doctor as I knew without a doubt that many others might not have diagnosed such a rare disease as quickly. This pediatrician was great and truly cared about Kendyl, both before and after the diagnosis.

December 23, 2015

My mom and my in-laws went back home. It was hard to say goodbye again. Kendyl was still in the hospital, and it was so hard to comprehend what we were going through. It felt like we were in a bad dream, and I kept hoping that I would wake up from it, but that wasn't the case. If it hadn't been two days before Christmas, I think my mom would have stayed with us even longer.

The next week went by slowly. It felt a bit like Zach and I were living two different lives. We would joke that he was raising Alyx, and I was raising Kendyl. Each day would be the same. I stayed at the hospital with her 24/7, while Zach stayed home with Alyx. They would come to see us at the hospital for a few hours each day. Some nights, after Alyx was asleep, Zach and I would do a FaceTime call.

I remember being a little frustrated that it took a few months longer than anticipated for me to become pregnant with Kendyl. We later realized that she had come at the perfect time. Zach had three weeks off from school. That was the longest break he ever had during his three years of JD/MBA school. It was so nice to have him out of school for three weeks and able to care for Alyx while I was at the hospital. We still had a lot of support from neighbors and friends but having that long break for Zach helped so much. I know that God knows us and that He is present in the details of our lives.

God knew exactly when Kendyl needed to come to our family. He knew she would be born with this disease but that we wouldn't know it for over two months. He knew Zach would be in school. He knew she would need major surgery. He knew we didn't have family around. He knew the best timing to get through everything. He knew all of it. God always knows.

December 25, 2015

You never picture being in the hospital for Christmas. It was a challenging day, but I think the hardest thing was knowing that we could not follow our original plan to go home for Christmas and surprise our families. The anticipation of that moment was so exciting to look forward to. Instead, not only would there be no surprise, but we were in the hospital, had been given a life-threatening diagnosis, Kendyl was recovering from a major surgery, and we weren't even together as a family.

My heart was so touched as I woke up that morning and saw a red Little Tikes wagon full of toys. Both girls had gifts, including some of their very favorites. People are SO generous. At first, I felt guilty and wondered if I should try to hide the wagon, until I realized later that every kid had been given a wagon filled with presents that fit their gender, age, etc. Zach came to the hospital with Alyx, and we tried to make the most of the day. We watched Christmas movies together in Kendyl's room and took her on many walks around the hospital.

That day, we met a family who had a child fighting a very rare form of cancer. They had several other kids and they also mentioned that they lost one a few months after birth to unknown causes. They were the happiest people I had ever met, and I was impressed with their strength

26

and faith. They were so friendly and seemed to be the kind of people that genuinely enjoyed talking with people they didn't know well (unlike me). While Alyx was in the playroom with some of their kids, they began asking me questions, getting to know our story and me, and they were just so happy. I kept wondering, "Do they not realize what day it is and where we are?" As I got to know them, I soon realized their son's diagnosis was even scarier than ours.

I hope to never forget that amazing family that we met at the hospital on that Christmas Day. I learned a lot from them that day and I have been forever grateful for this happiness lesson to me and my family.

You can uplift others, even when your heart is hurting.

December 31, 2015

It was New Year's Eve, and we were finally discharged, after three long weeks in the hospital. I was SO excited to go home. I was nervous to take Kendyl home but done with the hospital life. I often found myself thinking about the events and what had happened in such a short amount of time … her blessing day, a doctor's appointment, a life-threatening diagnosis, a surgery. It was a lot to process.

Zach took Alyx to a friend's home and then came to get us. I was feeling some guilt as we packed up from our hospital room, knowing others weren't going home. It was humbling to see people who were staying in the hospital being genuinely happy for us and excited that we were going home.

Celebrate other people's victories,
even when you are still waiting for yours.

We arrived home and we began following Kendyl's treatment protocols at home. Zach called it "The Melaney Hospital." We were on a strict schedule with IV medications three times a day, her tube feeds, etc. but we were willing to do whatever we needed to do so we could have her home.

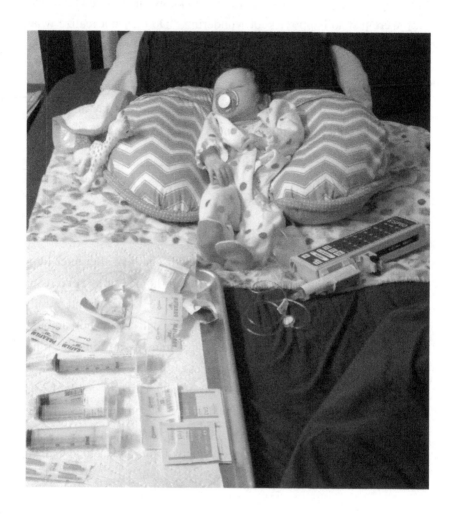

Chapter 2
LiveReal
2016

January 2, 2016

One advantage of holidays with little ones is that they don't know what day it is. Because of this, Zach and I decided to postpone Christmas until we could be together. We spent a few hours at the hospital together on Christmas Day but waited until we were home to celebrate. When we returned home on December 31st, after being in the hospital for three weeks, and having one good night in our own beds, we decided it was time to celebrate. We adapted to Kendyl's medication schedule and felt more comfortable with it.

For us, this was our Christmas Day. It was a wonderful Christmas morning and day together. We had FaceTime calls with family, and they all went along with our Christmas celebrations. Alyx had no idea, and this meant a lot to us. I was so grateful that I had listened to the feeling that I had to be ready for Christmas early.

January 2016

I was sitting at church one day when a sweet older lady came up to me and told me that she had been an ICU nurse for over 20 years. She was aware of Kendyl and asked how she could help. My immediate response was "Oh, thank you! That is so nice of you, but we are doing OK." This was a typical response from me as I did not ask for or accept much help. However, she kindly insisted she wanted to help.

She came later that week and could not have been any sweeter. She would often come to the house and tell me to go somewhere. I would laugh and respond with, "I don't really know where to go." She would tell me, both firmly and lovingly, to get out and take a break. When I would return home, I would find Kendyl peacefully asleep in her arms as she was rocking her back and forth. It was so comforting.

She helped us for several weeks. I was so touched that she not only asked how she could help but also didn't let me off the hook. This was a powerful example of not just saying, "let me know what I can do to help," but of showing up to help.

What can you do today to help someone else?

January 2016

I believe we all grieve differently. I remember going to Target with Kendyl a few weeks after everything had happened. I found myself just crying as I walked through the store. I tried to keep it together, but the tears were flowing, and memories kept coming back of the last time I was there with my two healthy girls, or at least that's what I thought. Kendyl was sick at the time, but we had no idea, so in my mind everything was great. No one in the store could possibly imagine why I was crying, and I didn't want to talk about it, but for me it was a way of grieving. I found myself going through this over and over. Each time I visited a store, I found myself thinking, "last time I was here everything was OK... I had no idea my life was about to change forever."

Give yourself time to grieve. People around you are loving and they care, but they don't know exactly what you are going through. Even if they try to sympathize with you, there is no way for them to know.

Everyone grieves differently. Be patient with
yourself and others during times of grief.

January 12, 2016

It was Zach's birthday and Kendyl had a doctor's appointment. A sweet friend came to babysit Alyx for me and I was hoping that she could do me another big favor. I asked her if she could make Zach's birthday cake. We both laughed but she happily agreed. I really appreciated it. I knew Zach didn't care much about his birthday and wouldn't have made a fuss about not having a cake, but I cared, and I wanted to have one for him. I was grateful we had a cake that day, even though it wasn't exactly the way I had imagined it. For years, Zach and I have laughed when remembering that this sweet lady in our neighborhood made his cake that year. It is good to be flexible about how tasks can get done.

January 24, 2016

We had been home from the hospital for a whole three weeks (the same amount of time we had been in the hospital), and it felt like we were just getting into the rhythm of things. We had celebrated Zach's birthday and a week later Alyx's birthday and life seemed to feel a little more normal. It was a regular Sunday, until I went to change Kendyl's diaper and noticed her stool was gray. No color, which we knew was NOT a good sign. I tried not to panic but at the same time I knew what this meant, and I knew it wasn't good. I called the nurse and sent her a picture of it. She told me that Kendyl needed to get blood work.

The nurse came to our home, drew blood and said she would be in touch. A few hours later she called me. I was on the phone and trying to stay hopeful until I heard her say 3.2. I still remember standing in my office, where it was quiet, and staring at that number I had written on a piece of paper. Normal bilirubin for children is less than 1. At her last blood draw, her bilirubin number was already higher than we wanted it to be at 2.9 but this jump in the wrong direction was not good.

After getting in touch with the G.I. doctor, the nurse called back and told us to go to the ER. I called a neighbor to come over and sit with the girls while Zach helped me pack a bag. We dropped Alyx off at another neighbor's house and left for the hospital. I couldn't believe we were back already. I just kept thinking, "This can't be real," or "Is this what life will always be like? In and out of the hospital?" My mind raced as she was admitted.

There is good and bad in every situation, but you have to look for it. It was easy to see the bad in the situation but as I took a step back, I was so grateful we were able to celebrate both Zach and Alyx's birthdays with Kendyl home.

January 2016

As our hospital stay continued and the days went on, we worried about Kendyl's future. There was a lot of testing and blood work. It was an emotional roller coaster each day to get blood work and then wait for results. We would hang on to those numbers and celebrate when they would go down and feel discouraged each time they went up.

We were blessed to have an amazing doctor who truly cared, Dr. Z. She would have me keep some of Kendyl's diapers and each time she would come to visit her in the room, she would look at them for color and signs of what her body was doing. Even as her mom, looking at diapers was something I didn't want to do. I was amazed that this doctor cared enough to do this.

One thing that was interesting to learn was that the smell of diapers matters. Bile makes diapers stinky, but when your body isn't releasing the bile, there isn't much smell. This was the case with Kendyl. It was the first time in my life when I began to realize how important dirty diapers were. Appreciate the stinky diapers of little ones. It means they are healthy.

January 27, 2016

We were still in the hospital and things weren't going as well as we had hoped. Kendyl was recovering well from surgery, but her bilirubin was still high and didn't seem to be going down much. We tried to get firm answers from the doctors. Although they kept telling us to be patient, we felt that there was more going on than what they were telling us.

While we were in the hospital, the team of doctors arranged for us to meet with a surgeon from the Seattle Children's Hospital. At the time, our current hospital didn't perform liver transplants, nor did any hospital in the city. The Seattle hospital was about four hours away from our home in Spokane.

When we met him, he pushed on Kendyl's belly and mentioned that he could feel that her liver was hard, and she would need a transplant. He didn't really mention when, yet he was very confident that she would need it. We asked many questions but also held strong to our belief that she wasn't going to need it anytime soon. In our minds, organ transplants seemed like something for other people, but not us; it just felt so unrealistic. That hospital was too far away. How would we do that? We thought for sure that our prayers would be answered, and that Kendyl's Kasai surgery would last her several years.

January 28, 2016

I had been very lucky to have family with me every time Kendyl needed a procedure, even though they lived 700 miles away. They were constantly coming to Spokane to help, and it truly meant the world. One day, Kendyl was going to have her PICC line removed because it was infected. (A PICC line is a thin, soft, long tube that is inserted into a vein. The tip of the catheter is positioned in a large vein that carries blood into the heart. It is used for long-term intravenous antibiotics, nutrition or medications, and for blood draws.) It was a very minor procedure, but I still didn't like the idea of going by myself as Zach had to go to school. I told my mom about it on the phone, and she suggested that I ask someone to go with me. I debated about it all day and didn't know what to do. I really hated asking people for help. It's always been hard for me. I like to do things on my own and I would much rather help someone else than ask for help but I couldn't change the situation I was in.

Kendyl had a very sweet nurse that night, so I felt comfortable leaving to get some sleep in my own bed. After a few days, that was welcomed. When I got home, I finally called a friend from church and asked if she could come with me. When I told her that we would need to leave at 7 a.m. the following day, I heard some slight hesitancy. I started to say, "It's OK don't worry about it." However, she reassured me that she was happy to help.

That next morning, she picked me up and we went together to the hospital and everything with the procedure went well. In fact, by the time I was able to see Kendyl, she was alert and playing with toys. My friend was the perfect person to be there with me that day. She was funny and I really needed some good laughs. She was also curious about Kendyl and didn't know too much about what was going on. My friend asked questions which gave me a chance to talk and process things. She was thoughtful and gave me compliments that really lifted me up. I had asked her to come for just a few hours, but she stayed with me all day. It was something that I will never forget. Although she was willing to help, she would have never known of my need that day if I hadn't asked.

There are times when people don't know what is going on so we must ask for help. If I had not asked, that day would have been much more stressful, and I would have missed out on spending time with such a wonderful friend.

Don't be shy to ask for help when you need it.

January 29, 2016

My mom came out to visit again. This time she wasn't sure how long she would stay so she bought a one-way ticket. I know it was hard for her to be so far away from us with so much going on. All her trips to Spokane were not only hard on her but also on my dad. It was also hard on my sisters and niece who still lived at home. It was a sacrifice for all of them and I will forever appreciate those sacrifices.

34

I didn't know it at the time, but the timing of this trip was absolutely perfect and just what was needed. I truly believe God had his hand in the timing and planning of this trip.

February 2, 2016

Today was one of the worst days of my life. After watching my little baby go through a major surgery and healing, we heard the dreaded news that I prayed we would never hear. The room was full of doctors, nurses, and social workers when we heard the words "Her Kasai has failed." It's weird how in some ways I was shocked but in other ways I was expecting it. I felt like they weren't telling us everything for a few weeks after her surgery, so I just kept hoping. To make things worse the surgeon who had performed the surgery had retired and we now had a different doctor. We immediately missed the gentleness of the first surgeon. The words the new surgeon said that day pierced my heart. "Just go home and enjoy your baby. This is the best time you will have with her."

What? I had just been through hell over the last few months watching my baby suffer. Are you telling me that was the best time? That I should enjoy this time? I was heartbroken, furious, and felt so many emotions at the same time. We then started to wonder what we were going to do. How could we keep living like this? I couldn't be in two places at one time. I couldn't care for Alyx and be at the hospital each day with my baby. Zach was busy in school and although he wanted to just quit at times, we knew he couldn't do that. I still admire how he kept up on studying while our lives were in complete chaos.

I'm grateful my mom was in town and at the hospital when this news was delivered. I was completely devastated. I felt so overwhelmed and heartbroken. I felt helpless. I felt lost.

Always have compassion. In many situations, the important thing is not what you say but how you say it. This was truly devastating news and there was no happy way to say it. However, the way it was said was cold, straight to the point, and so heartbreaking. It was hard enough to hear the words but the way it was delivered just broke my heart.

Show compassion to others even
when hard things need to be said.

February 2016

A few days after we learned that the Kasai procedure had failed, my mom suggested that the girls and I should consider moving back to Utah. Again, it was a weird feeling because I immediately thought, "No! There is no way" and at the same time it felt so right. Zach had a lot of stress with school, and it was hard for him to be there for us. Alyx was being taken care of by different neighbors and although she was having a great time, it wasn't a good solution in the long term. I was with Kendyl most of the time, wherever she went. Being in and out of the hospital with not much notice was also hard. I wasn't quite ready to say it out loud, but deep in my heart I knew that it made the most sense to move back home to Utah instead of moving to Seattle where we had no family. I knew this was something we needed to do, even though it wasn't what I wanted to do.

After we took in the news that Kasai had failed, we started discussing a liver transplant. I recall every meeting I had with doctors or nurses as I just sat there trying hard to pay attention. I just felt this couldn't be real. My baby was going to have a transplant? This isn't something I had pictured in my life at all. I knew nothing about transplants!

Not only did it feel scary to move away from the hospital and leave Zach behind, but it felt so scary to fly with Kendyl. Although she didn't look that sick, she was ultimately flying in preparation for a transplant. It was the only time in my life when I really wished I had a private plane or knew someone who did. We even looked to see if there was some sort of medical flight she could take but she didn't qualify for it. It was hard to think about taking her on an airplane when we had been so careful to keep her away from people and germs. We still knew it was the best option.

The decision to move was so sudden! My sweet sister had planned a trip to come to Spokane to visit and meet Kendyl in February. She even had her plane tickets booked, so she had to cancel everything when our plans changed. I knew in my heart it was the right thing to do, there was no doubt in my mind. It was so hard and definitely not what any of us wanted or would have chosen but that was the situation we were in. We moved forward and prepared for the move, wishing there was something we could do to change it.

Even though a decision might be right,
it doesn't always make it easy.

February 7, 2016

It was Superbowl Sunday, a fun day for most. I knew I needed to go to church and feel the peace there. It was the first Sunday of the month, which meant that the meeting was open for people of the congregation to share their testimonies. I was an emotional mess that day and even carried a small box of Kleenex from the hospital with me. I didn't even think about it until the person speaking after me mentioned that he recognized my Kleenex from the hospital. Although I hadn't planned on getting up that day, I bore my testimony of faith in hard times and the message that God is always there for us, no matter what we are going through.

After church, I immediately went back to the hospital. Although we had tried to avoid it, we agreed with the doctor to have Kendyl get a NG (nasogastric) feeding tube, and it was now time for this. She wasn't eating much or gaining weight, so they advised this would be the best thing for her. It was awful to stand outside the door and watch two nurses put the tube in while hearing our daughter scream. It hurt my heart and was so hard to watch. I told myself that I would never be able to do that on my own. (Little did I know then, it wouldn't be long before I would be doing it by myself, and I would sadly become quite good at it.) I picked her up and snuggled her right after it was placed. I couldn't help feeling sad to see this tube and tape covering her beautiful face. Sadly, it was something else we would soon get used to.

A few hours later, our Stake President (a leader of multiple congregations), came to visit us. He brought such a sweet spirit and apologized that he didn't know what had been going on (we didn't blame him because he was the leader for so many people). I found it very thoughtful of him to come on Superbowl Sunday, when he most likely had plans to enjoy the game with his family and loved ones. But he put our needs above his own desires (a true measure of a great leader). Although he was very focused on us, we noticed him glancing over at the score a few times, which was totally normal in the circumstances. It got me wondering what kind of party was going on at his house while he was with us. I was grateful that he would come visit us when I'm sure he would have loved to be at home with his family, eating yummy food and watching the biggest game of the year.

Before leaving, he offered a powerful prayer. It was long and while I don't remember everything, I do remember very well how I felt. I was at peace and knew that God was aware of us and our exact situation in every detail. We knew he was an amazing church leader and felt that he loved us, even though he didn't really know us well. I also clearly remember when he said something like, "I pray she will be healed quicker than anticipated." I was shocked when he said this. I clung to those words for years and although I was skeptical, I prayed that he would be right. That act of service, of coming to see us, stands out vividly in mind. We will never forget his selfless service that day and will forever appreciate it. The prayer he said did come true, but it was years later. I was expecting a faster result after this beautiful prayer, but it did come.

February 10, 2016

People around me tried to make it a special day on my birthday, even though Kendyl was still in the hospital. My sweet friend brought balloons and we had lunch in the cafeteria. My mom also wanted us to go do something fun that evening. She stayed with Kendyl at the hospital while some of our friends watched Alyx. Zach and I went to dinner and tried to keep it together, but it was hard. Our world was collapsing around us while others were living life to the fullest. It seemed so unfair. I don't know if we had never paid attention before, or if it was just that night, but we noticed so much coughing nearby. It really annoyed us knowing that we now had a daughter who was sick and who would never be completely normal because of her immune system. We became a lot more sensitive to this. Even though our lives were crazy, it was still good for us to get away and make the most of the day.

February 11, 2016

Kendyl was discharged from the hospital. What a roller coaster! It started in December with a 3-week hospital stay (including surgery), 3 weeks at home, and another 3-week stay in the hospital.

I was so ready to go back home and start packing up in preparation to leave for Utah. I was anxious and wanted to spend as much time with Alyx as I could before she would leave with my mom. When leaving the hospital, I thought to myself, "OK. We only have to make it one week." That's when Kendyl and I would be leaving, and I was determined to keep her home and out of the hospital for that long.

February 13, 2016

My mom and Alyx were leaving to fly to Utah. It was a cold day, and Alyx was wearing her black sweater with gold hearts and her cream-colored pants. She looked so cute that I took her outside to get a picture on our front porch. I wanted to get the most perfect picture to capture the moment. It was hard to hold it together and be strong, but I had to be brave for Alyx. I had never been away from my little girl for a long period in her whole life, so it was so hard to know she would be in a different state. It was also hard she was not understanding what was going on.

We knew it would be best if she didn't fully understand. While she just thought it was going to be fun flying to grandma's house, in the back of my mind I wanted to say, "Honey, please remember this house, as you won't be coming back. Remember the memories you have made here and the friends you met. Give your daddy a big hug because you won't be seeing him for a while. And be nice for Grandma." I could not believe our Spokane adventure was ending like this! But I just kept that for myself and told her that I loved her. I wanted to know so badly what she understood and what she was thinking. However, I also thought it was a blessing that she didn't really seem to know or care. Yet I knew, and it broke my heart.

I was so grateful for my mom being with us and flying with her. I can't imagine what it was like for her. Not only was she flying back home with a 3-year-old granddaughter that she didn't plan on bringing back, but she would become her immediate caretaker for at least a week until I got there. She was also leaving her daughter, son-in-law, and sick granddaughter behind during a heartbreaking time. I was comforted to know that she was flying back where our family was waiting for her. While I knew that they would all be there to help her, the responsibility would mostly fall on my mom's shoulders.

As my mom and Alyx got seated on the plane, Alyx very calmly looked up at my mom and said, "Grandma, the plane is going to crash." My mom quickly comforted her and said that everything was going to be OK. My mom quietly thought that a crash would be par for the course we were on. About 30 minutes into the flight, when the plane hit some intense turbulence, she really began to worry if maybe Alyx was right. After all that had happened over the last several months, it now seemed as if it might be possible.

Luckily, the plane landed smoothly, and they both arrived safely. My dad and sister picked them up at the airport. I absolutely love a picture of cute little Alyx that was captured while she was running to my dad. She had a big smile on her face and was so excited to see Grandpa, while my poor mom was walking behind her with lots of bags. I am forever grateful for my mom taking Alyx home, for coming without a return date and for how the whole trip played out. The last few days turned out differently than anyone could anticipate, but exactly how it was meant to be.

I often think of this experience and how Alyx was just excited to fly with Grandma. That's what she focused on. The reality was a lot more complicated than that, but that's all she knew and could understand and that was a major blessing.

Sometimes it can be a hidden blessing to not understand exactly what we are going through.

After dropping Alyx and my mom off at the airport, I hung around a few minutes to pick up my grandma. She had already planned this trip to come see us some time ago. While she knew that we had made the decision to move, she still wanted to visit and fly back with Kendyl and me.

I was truly blessed to have so much help from family. I know it wasn't easy for them to travel back and forth (my mom and in-laws made several trips). I will forever be grateful for their sacrifices. I truly don't know what we would have done without them.

February 14, 2016

It was Love Day, aka Valentine's Day, and I was sad to not have my girls together. I wasn't big into taking cute pictures of them dressed up for holidays, but the fact that I didn't have the option made it harder for me. I missed Alyx so much! I took pictures of Kendyl, but it wasn't the

41

same without both of them together. The day of love left me feeling lonely and sad. Knowing that I would be leaving Zach soon didn't help. I received pictures of Alyx and knew she was safe and having fun with cousins. This meant a lot, but it was still a sad day for me.

Holidays can often be harder when you are going through something challenging or after the death of a loved one.

Be sensitive to those around you. Even simple
holidays might make people feel sad.

February 2016

Life is interesting and usually works out exactly how it should, although very differently from the way we might have planned. After making the decision that the girls and I would move to Utah, I reached out to the sweet older lady that had been helping us. (She also called frequently to check in with us to ask how Kendyl was doing.) We thanked her for all she had done for us and let her know we wouldn't need her help anymore.

As we updated her on our plans to move to Utah, she told us that she had been wanting to get into foster care but that it was taking a while and she couldn't figure out why. She said that things were now finally coming together, and it all made more sense. I was so touched and grateful when she told us that she believed it was meant to be this way, that she was supposed to help us and that's where she needed to be for a while.

Things really do work out. It might not always be the way we want or on our time frame, but they do work out. Sometimes it is so hard to understand why things are taking longer than we want, are harder than expected, etc. but there is always a reason.

February 18, 2016

I needed the car today, so I took Zach to school and left Kendyl home with my grandma. I took a picture as he walked away from the car and cried by myself for a minute as it would be the last day that I would take him to school. As we shared a car for the last three years, whenever I needed to go somewhere, I would take him to school and later pick him up. Today was the last day I would be able to do that. Suddenly, I was sad that I would no longer have the opportunity to do this small task.

My grandma and I then took Kendyl to her pediatrician for her 4-month check-up and to get her vaccines before leaving Spokane. It was so weird to be back in that office. All the eerie feelings of our last visit came flooding back. What an eventful two months it had been. She had woken up that morning with a stuffy nose and I hesitated about giving her the vaccines, fearing that she might have a fever and get admitted. While deciding about the vaccines, they took her blood work to make sure it all looked well before leaving. Her GI doctor was called, and it was decided that we would give her the vaccines. We got this over with (it's never fun to watch the little ones be poked) and headed home to prepare for our departure the next day. I still remember the appreciation I felt when saying our farewells to her pediatrician. I was so grateful that she discovered Kendyl's condition; that she caught such a rare disease.

We came home and I was frantically packing and preparing to leave. It was hard to concentrate. I was not only leaving, I was moving! It was hard to know what I would need until Zach would move back home. A few hours later, Kendyl's GI doctor called to say that her blood work was elevated, and she would need to be admitted. I couldn't believe it. We were leaving tomorrow!

For a little bit, we thought that we might need to change our flight. However, we were reassured that they could start Kendyl on antibiotics that night and give her another dose in the morning, and then she would be good to go the next day.

As I was about ready to leave to take Kendyl to the hospital, a friend showed up to say goodbye. I hadn't seen her in a while because of the time I had spent in the hospital and when I saw her, I couldn't keep it together and just cried. She had been one of those friends that the second I met her, I loved her. She was full of personality and fun and I had learned so much from her. We also ran together often before Kendyl was born and I loved that time we spent together. I was grateful for the timing of her visit and for seeing her before I left.

We arrived at the hospital and Kendyl's IV was placed right away. I stayed until the evening and before leaving, I got her in her pj's, settled for bed and wished her goodnight. I was so sad to leave her 'alone,' something I didn't do often, but I wasn't ready to leave the next day and I really needed a good night's rest in my own bed (assuming I could sleep). I kissed my girl goodbye and told her that I would be back tomorrow to pick her up. The sweet nurses were excited to love on her one last time and that brought me peace as I left her there for the night.

I was absolutely exhausted when I arrived home that night, physically, mentally, and emotionally. It had been quite a day. As I walked in my house, I noticed something on the porch. It was a book full of pictures and notes from my friends from church. I was instantly sobbing as I looked through every picture and read each note. I was so touched by their kind words and knew I would treasure it forever.

It was a hard day but one full of tender mercies that came at the perfect time. Years later, I still treasure that book. It was such a thoughtful gift which reminds me of all the amazing people we met while living in Spokane.

Thoughtful gifts are the best gifts.

February 19, 2016

It was the big day. Kendyl and I were moving back to Utah. I felt conflicted, going through so many emotions. I was excited to be with

Alyx again. I was at peace knowing we were doing what was best for Kendyl. Yet I was so heartbroken to be leaving Zach, Spokane, and our little home we loved. I was grateful for our family opening up their home to us. It's hard to describe all the emotions I was feeling.

A few days before we left, a package with cute sweats arrived from my sister-in-law. It was so thoughtful! I was especially touched because she recently had a little baby. For her to think of me during such a busy time really meant so much. It sounds dumb, but I've always cared way too much about my outfits and considering all the stress, worry and heartache I was experiencing, it felt good to know that I was wearing cute and comfy sweats which made me feel loved.

Another family member, who had visited us and bought a Gonzaga shirt, sent me a picture of him wearing it that day to let me know he was thinking about us. It was a simple act, and yet I still think about it. I'm not sure if the family members remember these acts of service years later, but I do.

Zach drove my grandma and I to the hospital. We got everything ready for Kendyl to be discharged and said goodbye to the doctors and nurses who had taken care of her. It felt weird to say goodbye after what we had been through and knowing we weren't coming back. I was so glad to see one of my favorite doctors working that day so I could tell her goodbye. I really felt the sympathy and love from those who had taken care of Kendyl as we said farewell and thanked them for all they had done for us.

Someone in the hall who had seen us there a lot said, "Oh good you are going home." I smiled, as I tried to keep it together, and said, "Not exactly, we are being discharged to fly to Utah and get her ready for a transplant." The person looked at me in disbelief and you could see the genuine feelings of love and concern. Even though we were aware of the situation, it was still hard to take in. It didn't seem real and Kendyl didn't look that sick, even though her labs showed otherwise.

I sat in the back of the car with Kendyl on the way to the airport and my grandma sat in front. As we drove, I stared at my baby in her car seat. I couldn't believe we were leaving Spokane and the circumstances we were under. I knew that the time was approaching, as Zach was in his last semester, but I could never have predicted it would end like this and on such short notice. I thought of how I came to Spokane kicking and screaming and now I was leaving, kicking and screaming once again.

Zach helped get everything out of the car and walked us in. Spokane is one of the best airports because it's not busy, so he parked right in front for a minute and helped us walk in with our things. I gave him a hug and a kiss, and the tears flowed as I said goodbye. I couldn't believe the future we were facing and that he wasn't going to be with me for several weeks as we started this heartbreaking journey. I will never forget watching him tell Kendyl goodbye and then driving away. As sad as I was for me, I also felt sad for him. I can't imagine what it was like for him to tell us goodbye, knowing what he was going to miss, and trying to focus on finishing school strong while our lives were falling apart.

We went through security, something I had done several times with ease, but this time it felt like a disaster. TSA was giving me a hard time about Kendyl's formula that was hooked up through her feeding tube. They were trying to investigate the formula that was in her feeding bag and looked at all her meds and supplies I had with me. I tried over and over to explain the situation, the care that she needed, the reason we were flying to Utah, which was to prepare her for transplant, and that we wouldn't be coming back (hence the large number of supplies). Yet, they didn't seem to understand or care that much, and they continued to touch everything while I tried to explain that she was immunocompromised. I tried to keep my cool, but I felt frustrated. It was clear and easy to see that the formula was being pumped into my daughter at that very moment and yet they were still questioning why I needed the liquid formula.

It was a frustrating experience. I even had a doctor's note explaining the situation, but it didn't matter. We finally got through and I tried to erase the memories from my mind of them touching everything. I learned later that these types of situations can be much easier with TSA Cares. When you call ahead and explain your situation, you get more leeway for what you can bring, if it is health related. I wish I had known this before we traveled.

I was grateful that my grandma was there to fly with me. It was nice to have an extra set of hands. I can't imagine how I would have done it by myself in this situation and all that I was traveling with. As we boarded the plane, it was convenient that Kendyl had a visible feeding tube. I hoped that people would understand to stay away so she wouldn't catch any germs. When we got seated, we realized that we were able to keep her in the car seat between my grandma and me. This was a huge blessing to keep her in her seat and more shielded. It was a pretty easy flight, and I was so glad it was only an hour.

Salt Lake Airport had been home for so many years, yet it didn't feel like home. As we walked to the baggage claim area, I saw my mom. I tried to keep it together, but emotions were at the surface. She gave me a big hug and said, "how are you?" I said, "OK" as I teared up and she replied, "I'm so sorry." I know she was happy to see us, but the circumstances were heartbreaking. While walking to the car and passing people, a part of me wanted to shake them and say, "Do you know what is going on in my life?" Everyone seemed to just be going on with their lives like everything was normal. It felt weird that people weren't aware of my situation.

From the airport, we went straight to the hospital. It was quite a day to go from Sacred Heart Children's Hospital in Spokane, Washington, to the airport, fly to Utah, and go directly to Primary Children's Hospital in Salt Lake City. What a day!

I had talked on the phone many times with the doctor that we were referred to. As we were preparing to come to Utah, we had been told that that the hospital was ready for us. We became pretty well known at the hospital in Spokane because we were there so frequently and Kendyl was one of the only babies. She got lots of extra love and attention from the nurses. I assumed it would be the same experience at the hospital in Utah. However, as we got there, I didn't feel that was the case and I was frustrated. I'm sure it was because I was tired and everything was overwhelming, but our initial experience at the new hospital did not start out the way I had hoped for.

We finally got put in a room which honestly felt like a dungeon. The rooms were dull and small and the one we were in had no view. I honestly wanted to fly back to Spokane where I felt more comfortable. I knew most of the doctors and nurses after spending so much time there. I also loved their rooms. They were bigger and each one was painted a different bright and happy color. They had a big bathroom, and each room had a shower and a fridge. I had never noticed these things because it was all I knew until I didn't have it.

At one point it became too much for me and I started crying. My mom and grandma were trying to help but nothing they said could make me feel better. During my moment of tears, the resident doctor came in to introduce herself. I don't remember what was said but I was a mess and told her I didn't like this hospital. I probably wasn't very nice, but she listened, was very sympathetic, and asked what she could do to help. That resident ended up being one of my favorites.

My mom and grandma left late, around 10 p.m. I know they were both tired as it had been an exhausting day for everyone. After they left and Kendyl was settled to bed, I went downstairs to get something to eat. I was starving but found out that the cafeteria was closed. I went back to my room and laid on the couch bed as I cried myself to sleep with a growling stomach.

Change is hard. It's OK to mourn the past and want to go back to where you were before. It's normal to want to go back to where you are comfortable. But change is a necessary part of life.

We must be willing to accept change,
even when it's hard.

February 20, 2016

The next day was full of visitors from our family. It was nice to feel so much love and know that we were not alone. My sister also came to visit. I was so happy to see her as I hadn't seen her since the diagnosis. One of my husband's brothers came to visit as well. As we talked, he mentioned something that he hadn't told me before. He shared that when he came up for Kendyl's blessing in December, he didn't have a very good attitude. He knew that he would get home late that Sunday night and would have to drive for work early the next morning. When she was diagnosed and had the surgery, he realized how grateful he was to meet her that day, worrying if something were to happen to her. I was touched by his story and so glad that he shared it with me. I was grateful for family that came to visit that day and throughout the week. It meant a lot that even though Zach wasn't there, I knew I had family and support around me.

As the week went on, I felt better about being there and got more used to the hospital. I was able to meet the liver doctor that I had heard so much about. We had talked on the phone, but I now felt so much peace meeting with her. She checked Kendyl, pushed on her belly and said she thought it might be 12–18 months before she would need a transplant. I was relieved and joked that maybe we should go back to Spokane so we could be with Zach and come back when he graduated. Deep down I knew that we were where we needed to be, even though the change was hard for me. The hospital was different. The doctors and nurses were different. The rooms were different. It was a lot to take in.

February 2016

While we stayed in the hospital, I not only had to deal with the emotions behind moving and facing Kendyl's unknown future, I also had to handle insurance issues. We had been on state insurance in Washington (since we were poor students) and had now moved to Utah. It was difficult and overwhelming to do all the forms and paperwork to switch insurance carriers.

There was one day when it all seemed like too much and I was just crying in Kendyl's room. The social worker had come to visit, and I just lost it. In addition to everything I was dealing with, the last thing I wanted to worry about was insurance. She was very comforting and helpful and reassured me over and over that we would get things figured out. In a way, I felt like she held my hand through the process, and it was just what I needed.

While going through major situations, you often have to deal with things that most people wouldn't even think of, such as insurance. Let those around you help. I had no idea what social workers did before Kendyl's diagnosis and yet, both in Utah and Washington, discovered that they were so helpful.

There are resources and people ready to help.
They can often provide the guidance,
answers, and support that you need.

February 25, 2016

Kendyl was discharged from the hospital. What a whirlwind! We had initially planned to live with my in-laws but then they happened to get sick when Kendyl and I were coming, so we decided we needed to give them time to get better. We went to my parents' house instead and it was chaos with eight of us living together. However, I was so happy to finally have my girls together. I hadn't seen Alyx since she had flown to Utah because she had also been sick. She was finally feeling better, and I was thankful to be together again. Life still felt crazy as we started to get settled in a different state and place, but my girls were together. Things were a little bit more right in my world.

March 1, 2016

A week after leaving the hospital, Kendyl had a follow-up visit with her liver doctor. I was sitting in the back of the car with her, while my mom was driving us to the appointment. I couldn't stop staring at her cute face with a little clip in her hair, wondering what to expect from a clinic visit. It was a different experience because the first time we met them was in the hospital. This was our first visit to the clinic, and we would be meeting some of the team that I had spoken to on the phone. When they heard our names, they immediately recognized our story and knew that we were from Spokane. When we met the nurse practitioner, her first words were "I'm not sure how to say this, but I'm going to get right to the point. Kendyl needs be admitted." My mom and I were shocked. What? We had just taken her home. I really wasn't prepared to spend the night there. From that point on, I always had a bag in the car at every single appointment in case I needed to stay. Luckily, it was a short stay.

Always be prepared.

March 10–11, 2016

While most people in Zach's class were on Spring Break, going on fun trips to the beach or on cruises, Zach was driving from Spokane, Washington to West Haven, Utah. He drove about 700 miles to be with us for Kendyl's transplant evaluation, which would be done over two long days. This process included meeting with surgeons, nurses, coordinators, financial workers, social workers, and more. We covered what was involved with being listed, how much it would cost us for the transplant, what to expect with hospital stays, care after transplant and much more.

The first day, our families came with us. My parents, my in-laws, and my sister came to help with Kendyl because we knew she would probably be fussy and restless. We had gone through most of the evaluation before meeting with our social worker. As we all entered the room, the social worker told us that our families didn't need to stay. While we didn't mind them staying in the room with us, she told us that they weren't allowed to stay during this time. It was shocking to me; however, I soon realized why.

She asked us details from our childhoods, to growing up, and then to our marriage and how we deal with conflicts, problems, etc. Sadly, I started to realize there was more to a transplant than hospital stays and insurance forms. We began to grasp how much was going to be required of us. Having just the two of us with the social worker made it easier to answer questions without hesitation or judgment from family.

As we finished up the evaluation, I realized the importance of it and the reason it is so thorough. They really want to make sure that parents are going to take care of the organ that is offered. Otherwise, they want to give it to another child. Luckily, at the end she told us that we were going to handle this situation well and that she had full confidence in us. I felt like we had passed a really big test.

It was an exhausting two days. It was a lot, physically, mentally, and emotionally, to realize what was ahead of us. While it was sad that we were spending Zach's Spring Break this way, I was so grateful he could be there. The timing worked out perfectly so that he could be there without missing any days from school.

After the long evaluation, Zach drove back home. I can't imagine what was on his mind as he had over 10 hours alone to think about all the information, questions, and more.

March 18, 2016

Kendyl pulled out her tube again and for the first time I was able to put it back in myself. I needed help holding her down, but I did it. An NG tube goes up the nose and down into the stomach. It is awful and so sad. I also checked the placement by myself to make sure it wasn't in her lungs. I was so thankful it all went well and was comforted that I could do it by myself.

It's crazy to think that about six weeks earlier, when she had her first tube placed, I had told myself that I would never be able to do it. This was the first of many times. In fact, I became quite good at putting it back in because she pulled it out so often (even multiple times per day). Each time it broke my heart that I had to be the one to do it.

March 25, 2016

We were a little more settled in. I was living at my in-laws. That's a big statement by itself. But jokes aside, that was just a glimpse of it. I was living there without my husband, staying in what had been his room before we got married. Zach was the youngest of seven kids, and even though we had been married for almost five years, it was still known as "Zach's room." It was interesting to be there and share his old bed with Alyx and have Kendyl beside me in a crib, while Zach was in Spokane. It wasn't exactly how I pictured my life would be.

I was in that room when the liver clinic called me with good news. Kendyl was exactly six months old to the day when they told me that she was officially on the transplant list, and she had been listed with a PELD score of 13. I wasn't exactly sure what to say as many emotions hit me simultaneously. Feelings of excitement that she would hopefully receive a gift of life and feeling of sadness that she would get her gift through another child losing theirs. It seemed so unfair that there wasn't another way. I also had feelings of gratitude that I was an organ donor myself. This brought a flashback of the time I received my driver's license on my 16th birthday. At the time, most people in my family were not organ donors, but I couldn't deny the strong impression I had to become one. I felt strongly that was the right choice for me. As I got the call, I was grateful for the choice I had made years earlier. It made me realize the importance to make that choice before it's too late.

I wished so badly that Zach could have been with me that day. It was a lot to take in, especially since a month before, her doctor said she wouldn't need a transplant for 12–18 months. However, I appreciated that we were prepared. I was also grateful as I had no idea how fast and how sick my baby would become.

Sometimes, it might feel like we are going both forward and backward at the same time. That's how this experience felt.

Organ donation is an invaluable gift.
If you have not registered to be an organ donor,
please consider it. This could give someone
a second chance at life.

March 28, 2016

Zach had been able to come to Utah again for Easter. It was a great day to be together as a family. Even though it was a very short trip, we were grateful he could fly down and be with us. But it was a hard and tear-filled goodbye when he left.

As he left, I just kept telling him, "I can't do this. I can't do this." He would lovingly say, "Yes you can. You are doing great. Just keep going."

I truly felt that he meant it. He was saying everything I needed to hear, but I needed to hear it over and over. I needed to hear that I was going to make it through this hard time and that I was doing OK. I needed to hear that he believed it, as that would get me through the times when I didn't.

April 11, 2016

During today's visit at the clinic, along with my in-laws, the doctor mentioned that Kendyl was getting very sick. Dr. B mentioned the possibility of getting a liver from a different blood type. I was shocked as I didn't even know that was possible.

At one point, I asked why the doctor would mention a different blood type. When I said it, I felt I already knew the answer ... she was running out of time. Waiting for an organ that was the right size and blood type might not be possible or it might not come soon enough. The doctor never fully answered my question, but she said that she thought it would be a good idea so that she would get a liver sooner.

An organ from a different blood type can only be used with babies who have not yet developed the antibodies for other types, so the body won't reject it. Although I wanted Kendyl to get a liver as soon as possible, I hoped it wouldn't be this option.

My heart felt heavy on the way back home. My mom called a few hours later to ask about the appointment and when I told her the news, she asked me if I wanted to do this. I was thinking, "No, of course, I didn't want to." But I also didn't want to lose my baby girl. I had complete trust in her doctor and knew it was best to at least be open to this possibility.

April 18, 2016

Even though I had family all around me, I've never felt so alone. Even with all the help and support, it wasn't the same without Zach, especially during such a trying and stressful time. Living with family was definitely not the same as in my own house; I also didn't have my own car. Even though family on both sides were so willing to let me use their cars, it wasn't the same. I was always relieved when they came with me where I needed to go, and I didn't need to drive. It was one less stress that helped alleviate my heavy heart and mind. It is interesting to notice the little things you take for granted, and how you might not fully appreciate them until they are no longer there.

For a while, it was hard to describe our situation. Even simple everyday things seemed hard. I was at Costco by myself with both girls one day. Alyx was seated in the shopping cart with the groceries, and I had Kendyl in her stroller to keep her safe from germs that might be in the shopping cart. You can imagine how challenging it was pushing both around. This was a common occurrence because it was difficult to get out, so when I did, I would try to stock up on groceries to delay the next trip out as far as possible.

One time, I was approaching the cashier and saw a man with a few things in his cart. I asked him if he wanted to go in front of me. He kindly, and with a little bit of a laugh said, "No I'm good. I like watching you handle both kids." It might sound rude, but he didn't mean it this way. I laughed and told him to please pass in front of us, but he wouldn't.

I'm sure that if I had asked my family to help, they would have happily done it. They would have gone to the store with me or picked up the groceries. However, I am glad I that I often did this alone. It was a good learning experience for me. It showed me what I was capable of.

It is good for us to stretch. It is empowering
to know we can rise above challenges.

April 21, 2016

I was still living with my in-laws and Zach was in his last month of school when the company my dad worked for started laying off employees. They told him he could stay at the company and earn half of what he had been making before, or he could leave. Realizing the uncertain future of the company and having his salary cut in half, my dad made the difficult decision to leave the company. I was sad watching him go through it, and it felt so unfair with everything going on as well. I wondered, for a little bit, if God had forgotten about us. Were we not going through enough already? Why would this happen, and why now? I hate to admit it, but I was angry.

It took me some time to realize it, but the timing of my dad losing his job turned out to be such a blessing, and it was timed perfectly. I know that God had His hand in this, even though at the time it was hard to see, and I had questioned if He was even there and aware.

April 25, 2016

Kendyl had another liver appointment at the clinic. At this point, we were meeting with the team weekly. It was a one-hour drive each way. Those days would include lab tests, a clinic visit and sometimes other imaging; often we would also pick up meds. When that happened, the stroller was full. It was no small doctor's visit. Each visit would end up being a big day.

During this visit, we also discussed the findings from the CT scan from the week prior. This time, they found a few more things, the main one was that Kendyl's portal vein was really small. This meant that she would not be able to receive a liver from a living donor, so she would need a liver from a deceased baby. This broke my heart and Zach's as well. Zach had been hopeful that he could be the donor since they had the same blood type, but that was not a possibility anymore. That's when we also realized that Kendyl would have to get really sick before she could get a liver. When recipients get their liver from a living donor, they can often do surgery before they are too sick. Suddenly, this wasn't an option anymore.

Looking back, this was probably a blessing. I can't imagine what it would have been like to take care of both my baby and my husband at the same time.

Don't be afraid of hard news. The sooner you know,
the faster you can prepare and get through it.

April 30, 2016

My sisters-in-law took me to get a manicure and a pedicure so that I would have cute nails and toes for Zach's graduation. Since it was my first time, choosing the nail polish color was a big decision. It was nice to get out for a bit and have a little break while my mother-in-law watched the girls. It was relaxing to sit down without responsibilities and enjoy some much-needed laughs. They also took me to lunch afterward. It was a fun day that I truly enjoyed.

This was such a thoughtful gift. It wasn't only the value, but the time as well that I appreciated. It was something that I had never done and would have never done for myself during this time.

April 2016

April was a quiet month, in terms of hospital stays. It was the first month since Kendyl was diagnosed that she wasn't admitted. She still had weekly visits with her liver team, but no time spent in the hospital. It was wonderful!

Keep a journal of your life. Without it, you might not realize just how blessed you are or how far you have come.

May 2, 2016

It was the last clinic visit before I would be slipping away for a short trip to attend Zach's graduation (he didn't know I was coming). Since Kendyl was getting sicker, we were told at her weekly appointment that she had been approved for a score of 30, with an exception. (Scores are based on certain criteria, but if a doctor feels their patient is sicker than the score indicates, they can apply for an exception.) My mom was going to watch the girls while I went to Spokane. She couldn't believe that Kendyl's score would go up right as I was about to be leaving. We laughed thinking that a liver might become available while we were away and that my mom would have to take Kendyl in. Can you imagine what that would have been like for all of us?

The doctor also suggested placing a PICC line to start TPN (total parenteral nutrition, meaning through IV). This is a feeding method that bypasses the gastrointestinal tract. It allows fluids to be given into a vein to provide most of the nutrients the body needs. Since Kendyl wasn't tolerating her feeds very well, this was needed to help her get some much-needed nutrition. We hoped it would help her grow since she only weighed 12.85 lb and her arms and legs were so skinny.

Since I was going away, we decided to put it off for a week. Both my mom and I were relieved. We were told that because we were going to wait, we would put Kendyl on 24/7 feeds. This meant she would always be hooked up to her feeding pump whether she was awake or asleep. We hoped that she might tolerate her feeds better if they were given at a very slow rate.

May 6, 2016

I was lucky enough to be able to attend Zach's graduation. I will forever be grateful for those who made this possible. My generous father-in-law for flying me there, and my mom and sisters for watching my daughters.

I said goodbye to my girls before my mom drove me to the airport. I was nervous to leave them, but my mom was even more nervous to watch them. We joked again that she would get the call, even though I would only be gone for about 20 hours. (She didn't think it was very funny.) As I flew into the Spokane airport, I was nervous but so excited to go surprise Zach. He still didn't know that I was coming. I knew this airport so well from trips back and forth when I lived there. It was weird to be there by myself (I had only been there with one or both of my kids) and to reflect on what I'd been through since flying to Utah just a few months earlier.

My dad picked me up at the airport. I was so excited to see him. He drove to our neighborhood and dropped me off a few houses away so I could surprise Zach. He and my in-laws were finishing packing up our belongings.

I walked toward our house but after a few seconds I started running. I couldn't hold in my excitement as I ran to the home that I loved so much, anxious to see my husband. Zach was sitting on the porch after a long day of packing up the U-Haul and just stared at me as I ran up to him. It melted my heart to see his happy, surprised and smiling face as we embraced. He then laughed and said that when he saw me running, he thought to himself, "That girl looks a lot like Sam."

It was weird to see the house so empty. Zach, my in-laws, and my dad had worked so hard. I was grateful for all their help. It was an interesting experience to be moving without packing up my own house. This wonderful, little house that had truly been home for us, and a vacation home for family, would not be part of our lives any longer. Alyx was only nine months when we moved into this home. It was also where we brought Kendyl as a baby and where her journey started. This home had witnessed so many memories of our little family and many trips of family members visiting. It was hard to admit that we were really saying goodbye.

We locked up the empty house and headed to the hotel where we would be staying for the night. Zach had joked with my dad for months that the two of them were going to be bunkmates that night. Zach missed out on that, but I like to think me coming and surprising him was a little better. Everyone showered and got ready for dinner at Downriver Grill, a place I had always wanted to go to but hadn't been able to yet. It was a restaurant owned by someone we knew, and I had heard great things about it. The food was absolutely delicious, and they were so nice to give us some extra things to try on the house. It was a delightful evening. Of all restaurants we could have picked, it was the perfect one for our last night in Spokane.

I wasn't usually one to speak up about where to go to dinner or what plans to make, but I knew that I had wanted to go to this place for a long time and now was the best time to do it. I am grateful that I spoke up that night. We all enjoyed the food and our time together, but it probably meant the most to me. It was what I needed.

Don't be afraid to speak up.

May 7, 2016

We woke up early the next morning to get ready for Zach's graduation. I was able to meet a few of his school buddies before it started.

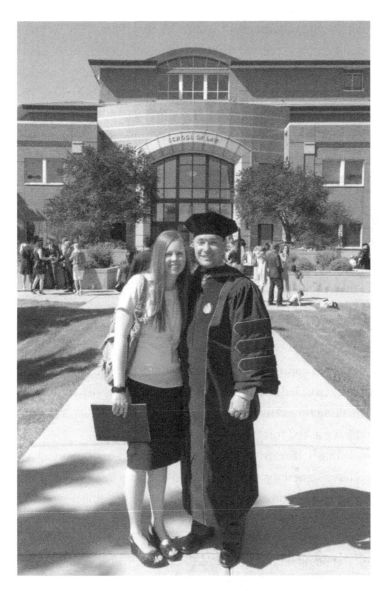

Zach went down with his class as we settled into our seats. As I watched him from my seat, I couldn't help but be amazed and so proud of him. I can't imagine trying to study while being a husband and a father, but especially during the last year when our life was so crazy. His commitment was amazing to me. When they called his name and I watched him walk the stage, my heart was full of love and gratitude for him and for the opportunity I had to be there with him. When I had moved in February, I feared that I would miss his graduation. I felt there was no way that I would be able to attend, and it broke my heart. I will forever be grateful that I was able to be there. That short 20-hour weekend trip was one of the best of my life.

After graduation, Zach and his father dropped me and my mother-in-law at the airport where we flew home together. There was no lunch or celebration; we were all anxious to get home. My dad started the 10-hour drive back in the U-Haul right away. When we landed in Salt Lake City, I was grateful and rejuvenated for having this little break. I was relieved to know that no liver offers had come in while we were gone, and all was well with my girls. My mom was brave to watch them, especially considering Kendyl's care and medications. I was relieved to be back home with them.

My dad is a champ and made an incredible time on the drive back home. He arrived home late Saturday night and Zach followed shortly after. It was so comforting to have Zach with us again. It had been very hard to be separated and even more difficult during such a stressful and heartbreaking time. His return was the best early Mother's Day present I could have asked for.

One thing I learned from this little trip is how important it is to always have something to look forward to. It can be something big, like a trip, or it can be something small, like shopping, dinner with a friend, a date with your spouse, etc. This can raise your spirits and bring you hope. Before leaving, when things got hard and I felt I couldn't keep going, I thought about how I was one step closer to the trip and celebrating Zach and his hard work.

Thinking about my trip, even though I knew it was going to be short, allowed me to push through the difficult days and kept me going for months.

Always have something to look forward to.

May 2016

Until May, I had mostly been living with my in-laws but after Zach arrived, we decided to move more permanently to my parents' house where we would have a little more space. We set up our "room" in the nook downstairs, all four of us. We had a queen-size mattress for Zach and me, a twin mattress for Alyx at the end of our bed, and a pack-n-play for Kendyl, right next to us on my side. We had her feeding pump on a stand next to the crib.

Our mattresses were on the floor, beside suitcases with some clothing for each of us, and no dressers. We made the best out of the situation, which we hoped would be short-lived. The house was full, nine of us to be exact! This included a terminally ill baby, a tired mom, a bar studying dad, a singing granddaughter, a recently divorced single mom and two-year-old daughter, a college student, a temporarily unemployed grandpa, and a worried and stressed-out grandma. It wasn't just the number of people living together that was difficult, but it was that we were all facing difficult life challenges. This was all happening while we waited for the "the call" that a donor liver was available.

It was a rough time, but none of us can deny the many miracles we experienced along the way. We joked that we were a re-enactment of the show Full House, which was our favorite when we were young. I really wish that I had a picture of our set up to remember that crazy time, but sadly I don't. At the time, we probably never thought there would come a day when we would want to remember it.

Take pictures. You can always delete a picture, but you can't go back in time to take one.

May 9, 2016

What a day! I went through some boxes of clothes and pulled out a few things for winter, just in case it took Zach longer to find a job and get our own place than we thought. I'm not sure what I was thinking, but when I packed a few things to move back in February, I kept telling myself, "Just get to May. Just get to May." It's a good thing that I didn't know how long it would end up being. It was a sad day as we moved all our belongings into storage. I had already been living with family for three months and it was just the beginning.

A few hours later, we had another clinic visit, but this time daddy was able to attend with us. It was so great to have him with us! There had been so many appointments without him, and I felt comforted to know he was here for good now and we could get through this together. During the visit, we discussed many things. We looked at that those who were on the list and their blood type. There were 5 with type A, 4 type B, and 14 type O, which was the same as Kendyl. It was discouraging to know that so many kids needed a liver from the same blood type. Originally, we thought that being type O+ was a good thing because it is a common blood type. However, we then learned that having many others on the transplant list with that same blood type would mean a longer wait. We also finalized plans to have Kendyl admitted the next day to get her PICC line and start TPN.

May 11, 2016

A day after Kendyl's PICC line had been placed, she was discharged to start TPN. A nurse came to the house around 10 p.m. to show us what to do. It was so overwhelming, and I just kept thinking, "I can't do this." There were two separate pumps and just like we had to do with the feeding pump, we had to prime the tubing so air wouldn't go into her

PICC line. It was challenging to carry her with both pumps (but thankfully they both fit in the same bag) and two tubes that were very short. I was grateful that Zach was back with us and that we would be handling the PICC line and TPN nutrition together.

May 16, 2016

It was becoming obvious that Kendyl's health was declining quickly. We had another day of labs and a clinic visit where we discussed the results. Her ammonia was up, her bilirubin was also going up, and we asked if TPN makes kids fussy since we had noticed Kendyl seemed fussier. We were told it depends on the child, and sadly that was our case. We also asked if she still needed to be on a specific vitamin called AquADEKs. She had been on it since the Kasai surgery, and it was awful. It was bright orange, stinky and stained all her clothes. Sadly, she still needed it and we needed to keep trying to have her take it and keep it down. It was a supplement with vitamins which we knew were important, but it was a challenge for us. We were also told to limit Kendyl's oral intake per day to 6 oz because her stomach couldn't handle more than that. It was important to make sure her meds would stay down. It was also important to continue to watch for fevers.

May 21, 2016

It had been about two weeks with the TPN, and we could already see a difference in Kendyl. Her arms and legs appeared a little bigger and she looked better and stronger. This was such a pain, but we were very grateful to see it was working!

It was an interesting experience to watch Kendyl around cousins about the same age (one being two weeks older the other five months younger) and yet they didn't look or act the same age. The cousins were normal, healthy, and thriving babies, while our little one was constantly hooked up to some sort of equipment (either formula through her feeding tube, or TPN nutrition through her PICC line, or both when the times would overlap). It was so sad. Instead of chasing a baby who would be rolling or crawling, I was holding my baby and pumps too. Between all the tubes, pumps and her growing belly, it was difficult to hold her. It was also hard to know how to keep her comfortable.

It often stung my heart a little to see them together, wondering what Kendyl would be doing if she felt good. I worried that if the worst happened, I might forever look at her sweet cousins getting older and wonder what she would have been like growing up. I was grateful they were healthy, and I couldn't help but wish the same for my baby.

Babies can be intimidating by themselves but when they are connected to equipment, they are even more so. I learned to be understanding when people didn't want to hold her. We knew it wasn't because they didn't want to, but it was intimidating for them to try. If you do want to hold a baby connected with equipment, please know it's not as scary as you might think.

May 23, 2016

Another day, another clinic visit. Today we signed papers to do a transplant study with multiple centers. We completely trusted the clinic we were working with, but we also knew that Kendyl was getting sicker. They recommended that we do this. We were also told to watch closely for fevers, bleeding, and an expanding belly.

May 29, 2016

Today was a good day. We were able to go to church together as a whole family. We had to leave a little early because a nurse was coming over to change Kendyl's dressing on her PICC line, but it was great to be there for the short time we were. We then had dinner with relatives visiting from Michigan, Louisiana, and New York, and with my sweet grandma who lived in a care center. My grandma was losing her memory and didn't really know who we were, but I was so grateful to see her. It was also a great opportunity to take a picture with her, which

I still treasure. This was the last time I saw my grandma before she passed away. It was also the last day Kendyl went to church for a long time.

When you have a sick family member, they need care and attention every day, even on Sundays. This was something new to me. I was always grateful when nurses could come to us instead of us going to them. Thankfully, home health is now available in many areas. I highly recommend it if you need help with a loved one.

May 31, 2016

We knew Kendyl's time was getting shorter. She had another doctor visit and we discussed why she might soon need to stay in the hospital. Internal bleeding, the need for daily monitoring and tummy taps are some reasons for hospitalization before a transplant. The team said the reason she was not staying in the hospital yet was because of the great care that we were doing at home. This was a very sweet compliment that really meant a lot to Zach and me.

Kendyl moved up to #7 on the waiting list for our region. Before they sent us home, they told me to watch for fevers and measure her belly each day to monitor if it was changing. As I watched her get sicker, I learned to be very observant. During this experience, I learned to watch for signs that could be overlooked if not looking carefully.

Being observant helps ourselves and those around us. Pay attention, even to the little things.

June 4–5, 2016

While getting her ready for bed, I noticed that Kendyl was breathing very fast and had subcostal retractions. This meant it was getting harder for her to breathe. It was a sign that we had been told to look for, so I started preparing to take her to the ER. My dad drove with me so Zach could stay back with Alyx.

After waiting for several hours in the ER, we finally got settled around 5 a.m. My dad stayed in the ER with Kendyl and me the whole time. I was worried about him driving home and kept telling him to go, but he wouldn't. Looking back, I appreciated that my dad could be there with us.

We woke up tired after a long night in the hospital. I'll never forget how Kendyl looked, with her tiny little legs and huge belly. It was obvious and sad that something wasn't the way it should be. That morning she had a minor procedure called paracentesis. This was done to drain the extra fluid that forms in the belly, a condition called ascites. It was the extra fluid in belly that was making it hard for her to breathe. Zach joined us at the hospital and stayed with me during the process. It was a minor procedure, but I was grateful that it all went well. We were also happy that she could have some relief from the drainage.

I had just gotten my girl to sleep and was about to lay down myself when the nurse came in. She told me that Kendyl was now an alternate on the list for a liver. There was another patient before her, but if something was found and they didn't feel comfortable operating on that patient, the liver would come to Kendyl. It was exciting, hopeful, and heartbreaking all at the same time. I immediately called Zach to let him know and he came down to the hospital. Luckily, we were now in a different room where two patients could stay at the same time. Since we had the whole room to ourselves, Zach and I could each have a couch bed. We sent a text message to our family to share the news. I had been feeling so tired but suddenly, I found it hard to go to sleep.

We knew that the probability was slim and that it would most likely not happen that night, but I still felt hopeful, knowing that my baby girl might soon be getting her gift of life.

I woke up a few times in the night when the nurse came in. Each time I asked if she had heard anything, and she would kindly reassure me that she would let me know if she did. Later in the night, the nurse came back and tapped on Zach's shoulder to let him know that the liver had gone to the baby on the list so our girl wouldn't be getting it. It was a letdown, but we felt happy for the family who did receive it and hoped that all had gone well. The next day Kendyl had a blood transfusion and then came home. This experience gave me hope. It gave me hope that her turn was coming too and that it might be soon.

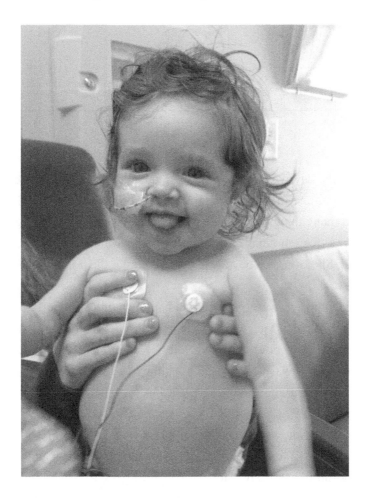

June 23, 2016

We had plans to go swimming at my in-law's new pool at night. As we were getting ready to go, I got a call from the liver clinic telling me that Kendyl was going to be an alternate for a liver again that night.

For a minute, I thought it might be better to skip the swim, just in case we got the call. After a few minutes, I decided to jump in the pool anyway and it felt so good. I was worrying about silly things like my hair but decided it would be fun to swim. The procedure was probably unlikely to happen anyway, and if she did get it, I could deal with my chlorine hair.

Live life to the fullest.
You will never get the moment back.

June 27, 2016

Most of the day was spent at the hospital. We had a long clinic visit, two chest X-rays, new stitches for the PICC line, and more blood work. We had many things to discuss again, such as getting her chicken pox vaccine a few months early so her body wouldn't be negatively affected. She wouldn't be able to receive it after the transplant because it is a live virus.

It felt like we were prepared and just waiting for the transplant, hoping she wouldn't get too much worse. I had to ask the hard question, "how much time does she have left?" I didn't really get a straight answer (which I wasn't surprised by) but was told by the team that they were, "confident about the transplant but prepared for a complicated surgery."

Kendyl was now nine months old. She was on TPN for 16 hours a day, lipids for 12 hours, feeds for 9 hours and lots of oral meds through her tube during the day. Her weight got up to 15 pounds and was officially in size 2 diapers. (She had been going back and forth between sizes 1 and 2 based on how big her belly was.) We were trying to stay positive and thankful she was still home with us. Her health was declining but it was comforting to know she was in such good hands.

I recorded in my journal, *"I look forward to the day when my little girl will feel good, when she won't be hooked up to so many pumps and*

when she can play on her tummy, move around, have more energy, and
eat real food by mouth. I look forward to the day she won't throw up all
the time and we can leave the house without packing up our lives."

July 10, 2016

This was it. We received the call that a liver was available for Kendyl.
We got everything prepared and packed, had a big family prayer, and
we were all so grateful that she was going to be getting her gift of life.
We had just gotten on the freeway when my phone rang. It was the
transplant coordinator telling us that the surgeon had changed his mind.
He had decided that the distance was too far and Kendyl would not be
having the transplant. We were devastated. It was at this point when
Zach told me that he feared she wouldn't make it. Our strong faith that
she would make it was dwindling. It was hard to stay positive after this.
We had so many questions with so few answers.

A setback doesn't mean never.

July 11, 2016

Kendyl had another appointment with the liver team. Her weight
reached 7.6 kg (almost 17 lb). Lab results looked OK, but some
numbers were concerning, including low platelets and high bilirubin (at
16).

We were getting a stronger batch of TPN, with more vitamin K, to
use each day. It was overwhelming! I felt like I could not handle
anything added to her daily care.

At this appointment, we also discussed criteria for a scary score
known as 1A and 1B. These scores indicated critically ill patients that
may not survive if they didn't receive a liver within 24–48 hours. It
includes patients on ventilators, with major bleeding, and those not able
to wake up. I prayed in my heart that we would never see this score. As

we left that day, we scheduled her next appointment for the following Monday, July 18th.

July 12, 2016

Kendyl had been throwing up again, which wasn't that unusual. However, this time I noticed that there was some blood, which was a sign that we had to watch for as it could indicate internal bleeding. I took a picture of the blood and called the liver clinic. They had us take her to the hospital to be admitted.

They told me that day she probably wouldn't be able to live at home much longer. Her care was getting harder, and she was becoming more fragile every day.

Most patients live in the hospital while waiting for organs, so I wasn't totally surprised. As I heard the news, I felt overwhelmed and heartbroken that she might need to stay there. How would we do this? How would I be in the hospital and care for Alyx at home? And yet, at the same time, I also felt a little relieved. I was really exhausted, and the constant care felt heavy, both physically and emotionally. I felt like it was too big of a load on my shoulders. We were told that she could go home the next day but that she would most likely be back soon to wait for her liver. We stayed overnight and came home the next day.

July 16, 2016

We stayed up later than usual the previous night. After the girls were in bed, Zach and I had ice cream and watched Dateline with my mom. (I had never really been into Dateline before, but really got into it during this time. In a weird way, it brought me peace when I felt that my life was out of control. It didn't feel quite as crazy when I watched that show.)

We hadn't been asleep that long. It was just after midnight, at about 12:15 a.m., when I woke up and realized I had missed a call from an unknown number. As I reached for my phone to see who had called, we looked at the number and recognized that it was the same that had also called the week before. We soon realized it was the transplant coordinator and this might be the moment we had been waiting and praying for. We barely missed the second call on Zach's phone as we were trying to be quiet with the girls right by us. A few seconds later my mom was running down the stairs and I then knew for sure who was calling. She handed me the phone and I went upstairs to finish the call and not wake up the girls.

They had a "perfect match." The liver was a B+ blood type, so while it didn't match Kendyl's (O+), it was compatible, and they felt that we should accept this offer. We told them we were on board, and they asked us to come to the hospital. We gathered our things and headed down to Primary Children's Hospital. We didn't let any other family members know as there wasn't much they could do, so it wasn't worth interrupting their sleep. We also knew we had a long day of preparation ahead of us.

When we arrived, I could hardly believe it. We went to our normal spot on the 4th floor which was the transplant/cancer unit. Some of the nurses remembered me and you could see and hear the excitement on their faces and in their eyes as we told them why we were there.

This was it! I could just feel it. The earlier experience when we received the call about a liver being available seemed way too perfect. But this time felt right since it was in the middle of the night, which is when these things often happen. They did hours of testing, there were SO many tests! They checked everything to be sure that she was healthy enough for the transplant. As the night went on, it got annoying because they kept coming in to poke her again and again. Each time she would start to go to sleep, they would come in again and repeat until they had everything they needed. It was hard to get her settled down when these interruptions would happen again and again. Around 4 a.m., Zach and I tried to get a little sleep. One of us was in the chair and the other was on the couch. It didn't last long, and we ended up not getting any sleep.

Between the worry and adrenaline, the chance of us getting any sleep was close to none.

For months, I had been wondering how this day/night would be and imagining my thoughts and feelings. I had visualized happy tears that she was getting her gift of life. However, as we sat in that hospital room, the emotions were very different than I thought they would be. We kept talking about the deceased donor and their family. We wondered how old the donor was and what had happened. We kept thinking of this heartbroken family and wondered when the funeral would be. I wished so badly to know the details.

As the night became morning, we slowly started letting our families know. Some came right away that morning as they wanted to see us and wish Kendyl good luck.

At around 2:00 p.m., they moved us to the ICU so they could do a procedure called Pheresis. This involves separating and filtering the blood and then returning a portion to the patient. It was done to remove the bile and clean the blood in her system to get rid of antibodies before her transplant. As we sat there and watched Kendyl hooked up to machines, we saw her blood separating with the bile taken out. When looking at the tube full of dark yellow bile, I kept thinking, "I can't believe that was in her body." It was amazing to see her skin and face color already changing. It gave us a peek at what she might look like after transplant.

As we got closer to the time of surgery, which was scheduled for 4:00 p.m., I started getting very cold. I was shaking and couldn't figure out what was wrong with me since I wasn't usually a cold person. They even brought me heated blankets and my mom explained that I might be in shock and that it was probably my nerves. Right before we took Kendyl to the operating room, I asked her doctor specifically how many other ABO incompatible transplants they had done previously. She told me three. I was relieved to know our daughter wasn't going to be the first, but I also felt a little nervous that it was such a low number. However, I knew it was right to proceed.

We said our goodbyes to our little baby. Here we were again, going through surgery number 2, a liver transplant. Kendyl would soon be receiving a full liver from a deceased baby. It was still hard to wrap my head around it. While it was such a happy event for her, it was still so hard to, once again, place her in the arms of the doctors and surgeons as they took her to the operating room.

For hours, we patiently sat in the waiting room. It was weird to have so much time on our hands but also not really be able to focus. I had books, my journal, and other things to keep me distracted but I couldn't focus. I was grateful that we had many family members waiting with us. It felt comforting to have their support and know we weren't alone. While sitting in the waiting room, I kept watching other families come and go. We enjoyed cinnamon bears that someone from our family had brought us while waiting for updates provided over the phone every few hours.

During the surgery, I wrote this post for social media:

"Little Kendyl has been in surgery for three hours so far. We got the call at 12:15 a.m. this morning and have been here since 2:00 a.m. We are exhausted and nervous but also excited. We are thrilled that she is having her transplant, but our hearts go out the family that lost their little one. We hope they will feel peace at this difficult time. We will be forever grateful they chose organ donation. We are grateful for Kendyl's wonderful doctor and team and their amazing care. We are encouraged by their words, "She is very sick, but she is strong." Thank you for all your prayers and concerns. We love you Kendyl Rose."

The surgery lasted about eight hours. Because it was very late, only Zach and I, our parents, and a few siblings remained in the waiting room. When we finally saw the surgeon come to the waiting room after 12:30 a.m., we couldn't wait to hear what he had to say. He told us that everything went well, and we would soon be able to see her. The surgeon looked tired but also satisfied. He told us he would be back to check on her in the morning.

When we were finally able to see her, we were amazed that she was off the breathing and oxygen machines already. She was still hooked up to many devices, but she looked good. We were so relieved! She was still asleep and would probably sleep most of the night. Although it was hard for me to leave her, we realized it would probably be a good time for me to go home. We had a long stay ahead of us.

Zach told me to go home while he stayed at the hospital for the night. He was in a PICU family room that we arranged before surgery. I went home with my parents and got settled in bed around 2 a.m. I had now been up for 26 hours straight. I remember feeling so exhausted, yet also awake, as I tried to go to sleep. When I finally drifted off, I slept deeper than I had in a very long time.

July 17, 2016

My dad woke me up around 7:30 a.m. the next morning. I couldn't believe that I had slept that late. I didn't mean to, but my body needed it. I jumped in the shower and then we rushed down to the hospital as I couldn't wait to see Kendyl. We got there right before the doctors did their morning rounds. The nurse said that she had a good night, and I was so relieved. I was amazed to see the team of 15 medical professionals all standing outside her door going through everything from the surgery. The surgeon said, "She had me work for it," meaning that it was a complicated surgery. Part of the challenge came from trying to get such a swollen, hard liver out of her tiny body. He also mentioned that the new liver was really small. My mind raced to know more about the liver and where it had come from, but they couldn't give us any information.

Overall Kendyl was doing well. We were so grateful that her yucky liver was out, and a new one replaced it. The first 24–48 hours are the most critical and we were feeling so grateful that she was doing well.

July 18, 2016

I was finally able to hold my baby girl. It was incredible to be able to hold her again. It took several nurses to help with all the wires that she was hooked up to, but they got us all settled. It felt so wonderful to be together again after such a procedure. Her big incision, which had the shape of the Mercedes logo, was impressive. I was worried that I might hurt her, but I was also happy and grateful to do it. My baby, not even a year old yet, had just received a liver from another precious little one. My heart was full of gratitude.

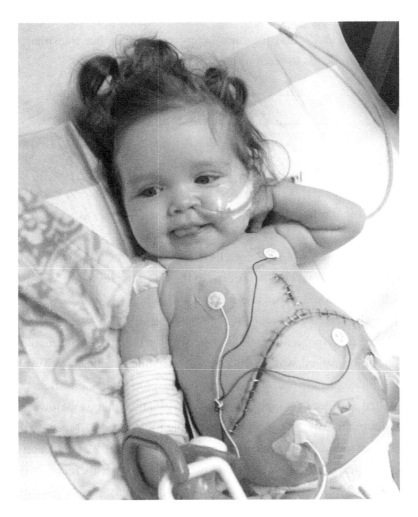

July 20, 2016

Kendyl was able to move from the PICU to her normal floor. This was a big deal and very exciting. Zach came to the hospital that day, as he often did, wearing his Kendyl Strong shirt. He was finally able to hold her for the first time since surgery. As I watched him hold her, I was overcome with gratitude, appreciation, and amazement for him. I can't imagine what he had been going through with school, finals, studying for the Bar Exam, etc. I truly felt so much love for him.

July 21, 2016

We saw Kendyl's first true and happy smile since her transplant. It warmed our hearts to see it return after a long five days.

Appreciate the little things.

July 22, 2016

It was nice to see both girls together as Alyx was able to come see Kendyl for the first time since the transplant. Alyx was so cute and sweet looking at her baby sister in her crib. I got to hold Kendyl again for a while and saw a few more little smiles. I also enjoyed being able to go with Alyx, just the two of us, to the hospital playroom. We spent quality time as we played and did crafts together.

Kendyl had to get a new PICC line but luckily, they were able to do it in the same spot and save blood vessels for the future. Her recovery after the transplant was very slow. She remained stable, which was a huge blessing, but she really struggled to progress. Soon after, they installed an Anderson tube in her nose. While this tube went down into her tummy, it was the opposite of a feeding tube. Instead of feeding her, it sucked out anything in order to monitor internal bleeding and to prevent her from throwing up. However, she was still regurgitating often. We couldn't figure out why because she only had IV nutrition, so there wasn't anything in her tummy. This was just one of the many hurdles she had after the transplant.

We had heard several times from the team that her surgery was very complicated and tougher than other transplants, so her little body had been through a lot.

There will always be hurdles along the way in life.
Try not to let them discourage you.

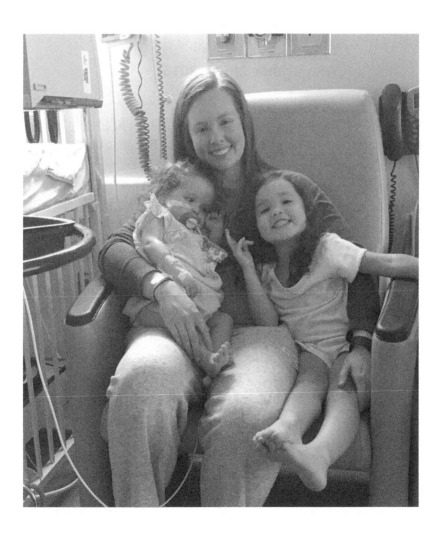

July 23, 2016

My mom, Alyx, my sister, and my niece came down to visit us at the hospital. My sister and I then took our girls to the Hogle Zoo while my mom stayed with Kendyl. We enjoyed a great day together! It was fun to spend time with Alyx and be out of the hospital for a bit. I was grateful for those who made this fun day possible.

I've often felt bad for what Alyx had missed out on because of her sister. One of the hardest parts of this journey was doing what was best for both girls and finding that balance. If you are in this situation, my heart goes out to you. Keep doing your best.

July 26–27, 2016

Ten days after Kendyl's transplant, while she was still in the hospital, Zach took the bar exam. I felt so bad for him that with everything going on, he still had to take the test. He studied the best he could, even with all the chaos in his personal life.

It took several weeks to get the results of his exam. He was very close but unfortunately didn't pass. I know he felt a little defeated, but under the circumstances, most would not have passed. I was still proud of him and the way he kept attending school and studying when our lives felt out of control.

I was mad when I heard he didn't pass. I felt that with everything going on, God could have helped Zach pass that test. We had been through so much and I wondered if helping Zach pass the bar was too much to ask. However, looking back there was a reason. After Zach got his results, we discussed if he would take the exam again. He went back and forth but decided not to and instead focus on getting a career that would use his MBA degree more than his JD. (Not to give it away, but he ended up in a field he never expected and absolutely loves! His salary and hours are much better than if he had chosen to be an attorney.) God always knows what He is doing.

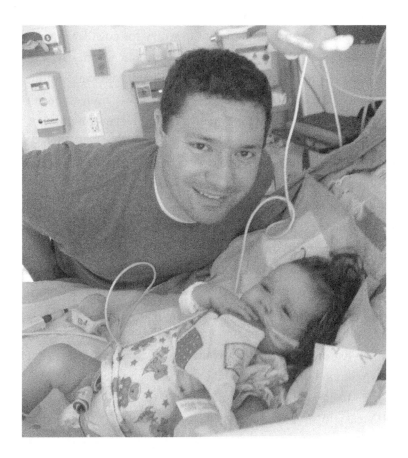

July 31, 2016

The team mentioned that Kendyl's labs were elevating, and this had been a trend for the last few days. My dad came to join me and we went to church together in the hospital, which was just what I needed.

Afterward, Kendyl had an ultrasound and a CT scan to look at the liver. Both results showed that her portal vein was clotted. It was hard to hear this only two weeks post-transplant, especially after everything we had been through. I had to keep reminding myself that it was better for the portal vein to be clotted than the hepatic artery. That would have meant a re-transplant ASAP.

I began worrying about this immediately after they told me (that's what I do best) but they told me not to worry for now. I was surprised to hear this but trusted them. Around this time, our amazing liver doctor introduced us to Dr. R., a wonderful surgeon who was visiting the hospital to see about joining their liver team. I was impressed with him and felt special that we were one of the families meeting him. It was mentioned that if Dr. R. joined the team, he would eventually be doing surgeries, such as fixing Kendyl's portal vein, as it was his specialty.

I felt so grateful for this team and especially with Dr. B., the liver doctor. There were other amazing doctors, but we got the best with the most experience. This was comforting to know since our girl was a such a complicated patient. I believe the best doctor in the field accepted her as a patient because we had been referred while we were living out of state. We had moved specifically near this hospital for her transplant and that was a big deal to the liver clinic. Even though we were technically moving back home where both Zach and I had grown up, the main reason for the move was the care she needed. Although it was overwhelming to even talk about another surgery, I trusted the doctor and tried to not think about the portal vein.

It's easy to stress and fear some situations, but if an expert in that field tells you not to worry, try to let it go. There is no need to begin stressing about something ahead of time.

August 2, 2016

We were about two and a half weeks post-transplant. I had taken a really cute picture of Kendyl and decided to compare it from the day when she was admitted to receive her new liver. I was shocked to see the difference. She looked like a different child and so much heathier. The color of her skin and eyes was so much better; even her hair was a little lighter. It is crazy to see what a difference a healthy liver can make. I was grateful I had taken the pictures so I could see the progress she had made.

It had been a rough week. We were reminded over and over that Kendyl had a very different anatomy than most and because the transplant was complicated, her insides had a hard time "waking up." She still had the Anderson tube sucking out her stomach and she was throwing up a lot. Because of these complications, she was still on TPN since she was not able to eat. I thought this would be only before transplant and never imagined she would need it after too.

I couldn't imagine what it felt like to throw up with her sore tummy covered in staples. She had a slightly better day and we hoped it would continue. At this point we weren't sure how long she would be in the hospital. Even with setbacks, we were happy that her liver was working and that her labs looked good. We saw her smile more, and we could hold her more easily. She also began to talk again. Kendyl continued to teach her mommy and everyone around her to be happy and patient, even when things don't go as planned. Although we had hoped a new liver would be a smooth transition, we were glad to be on this side of her journey and not still waiting for one.

It is easy to see how far you still need to go.
But if you take a step back, you might
realize just how far you have come.

August 4, 2016

Kendyl was slowly improving and started speech therapy. We tried a sippy cup that she seemed interested in but couldn't figure out how to use it. It was sad to watch a simple and easy thing, like a sippy cup, be hard for her. However, I was happy that she seemed interested in it and hoped that with time she would figure it out. Zach had given her a blessing to help her continue to heal and provide her with strength. Because the Anderson tube was not being used as much, we were able to get out of the room for a bit and go on a wagon ride. It was so much fun to be able to take her out of the room for the first time since the transplant.

My mom, grandma, and great-aunt came to see Kendyl along with my in-laws. We had a great time together, so I was sad when they had to leave. My sister also came visit and we were able to get dinner together downstairs in the cafeteria and then took Kendyl's 10-month-old pictures.

Before my grandma left, she kept insisting that I call to stay at the Ronald McDonald Room, so I could get a good night's sleep. It is on the 3rd floor of the hospital and has a big family area, kitchen, bathrooms, and sleeping rooms that can be reserved for parents. I felt I was fine, but she just kept persisting, so I called and was able to book one. Before leaving, I gave Kendyl her meds and as I was getting her to bed, she threw up twice. I completely lost it! I was so done with her puking and having to re-dose meds. My nurse was so great and told me to go and to get some sleep. I really appreciated having the room and a much-needed break. I was grateful for listening to my persistent grandma. The long stay was really starting to wear on me.

Don't let a whole day be ruined
by some unfortunate events.

August 2016

The days went on and I really got used to living at the hospital, and even doing my laundry there. This was something I had never even thought of and frankly didn't even know existed.

At some point, I began to notice that Kendyl's diapers were so stinky. I couldn't believe it. It was something that we had never really experienced. We laughed about being grateful for stinky diapers because it meant her liver was working and bile was being removed by her system. It's funny what you can become grateful for when you don't have it, such as laundry units in the hospital and stinky diapers.

What are you taking for granted,
which others don't have?

August 13, 2016

Kendyl was finally making great progress and was getting closer to coming home. It felt like we were finally almost there. They decided to give her a break from overnight feeds to see how her body would respond and get her used to not eating at night. She had been tube fed through the night for most of her life so I was worried that this might not be a good idea. I wondered if her body could handle this, but decided the doctors knew more than me and trusted them.

That morning, Kendyl seemed to be OK when they came to do her usual blood work but shortly after, I noticed that she was NOT herself. She was very lethargic and about the same time, the nurse came in to check on her and told me that her glucose was low. They checked her blood again and she didn't even cry or fuss, which made me nervous. Her blood sugar was 11, which is dangerously low.

They immediately began shaking her gently to wake her up … nothing. As I sat there by myself watching, I felt so scared. I wanted so badly for someone to be there with me but everyone from my family was about an hour away from the hospital. To make things worse, I couldn't even call Zach because he was taking the MPRE Exam (Multistate Professional Responsibility Examination, a test designed to measure knowledge and understanding for professional conduct working in the legal field). I called my parents. They answered and I didn't even know what to say but they could tell I was choked up. They told me that they would be on their way and to keep them updated. I felt a feeling of peace and knew that if anyone could get there the fastest, it would be my dad.

As I waited, I watched staff I didn't know come into the room after hearing about Kendyl's blood sugar emergency. They asked if I needed anything or if they could help. What meant the most was when one of the male nurses asked if I wanted a blessing. I didn't even know he was of my same faith, but I instantly told him I would love one and I was very grateful for his presence.

I already knew the situation was bad because of the way they were acting and the number of doctors present, but the moment I knew it was really serious was when I saw Kendyl's liver doctor outside the room. She came in specifically for her because she was nervous. When she walked into the room, I thanked her for coming and she said something like, "She has come so far, I just kept thinking we can't lose her now." It was both comforting and terrifying to hear those words. Looking back, I should have voiced my concern about turning off the feeds that night.

Always listen to your intuition.

August 2016

At times during Kendyl's stay in the hospital, Zach traded spots with me so I could rest at home and be with Alyx. Even though he wasn't able to do it very often, I appreciated it every time.

He stayed overnight and the next morning the phlebotomist came in for the daily routine labs. Zach picked up Kendyl to put her on his lap. After the phlebotomist prepared her orders, she reached for Kendyl's foot but accidentally grabbed him instead. Flustered and embarrassed, she quickly finished the lab draw and left as soon as possible. We never saw her again. While we feel bad for that sweet young girl, it is still making us laugh today. There was no point getting mad or flustered over this accident.

Life is short, so keep it light and choose to laugh.

August 21, 2016

I woke up feeling a little frustrated since Kendyl had had a fever the previous night and they didn't know why. The fluid of her drain was tested for infection, and it was clear. However, I was quickly reminded that it wasn't as serious as it could be. While I was meeting with the team for rounds, they had to run off to the PICU for an emergency. I couldn't help but think it was probably a post-transplant kid and how scary it would have been to be in that situation. I was able to take time to go to church and it felt so good to be there. I later met with the team again and they decided to stop the glucose checks (yay) and to stop both antibiotics which they thought might be causing the fevers. They also decided to wait on placing a PICC line.

Kendyl was able to play in the saucer for the first time since transplant, and I put her in one of her own outfits. My parents came to visit, and we were able to take a walk with the stroller. It was so great to be out of the room and even go outside for a bit.

August 23, 2016

After 40 days in the hospital, Kendyl was finally coming home! (It was actually 39 days but after being there that long it seems fair to say 40.) She had been close to being released a few times, but then something would always happen to set her back. We were so excited that day was finally here! We were thrilled as Zach loaded our bags. You can imagine how much we had accumulated over the weeks as I often brought more toys, books and other belongings while our stay got longer. I had stayed there the whole time except for a few weekends when Zach would switch with me. The nurses were so sweet as we left and were genuinely excited for us. They felt like family saying goodbye after such a long stay.

We drove home full of smiles and arrived at my parents' home where a big yellow sign said, "Welcome Home Kendyl." It was fun to see. I know that she was little and didn't really care about it, but I did.

She was wearing a cute and bright orange dress. Her feeding tube on her cheek had been freshly taped and I did her hair in cute pigtails. It was a big day!

I felt so much relief to be home. Technically, I still wasn't at my own house, but I was grateful to not be in the hospital. I appreciated having home-cooked meals and not having to do my laundry at the hospital any longer.

I'm glad we didn't know before the transplant that her stay would be that long. We had been told it would be about 14 days, which is the usual. I know that others have had longer stays and my heart truly goes out to them. But for us, 40 days was a long time and a lot longer than we had planned on.

For the record, Kendyl went home on 13 different medications— some were once or twice a day, while others up to four times daily. A few had to stay in the fridge while others didn't. It was a lot to keep track of, but it was worth it to have her home.

August/September 2016

After we got settled with Kendyl and more used to her care schedule, a friend of a family member offered us free counseling sessions. Zach and I had never been to therapy together but decided it might be good for us. At our first appointment, as we thanked him for offering to meet with us, he mentioned a heartbreaking statistic that 90% of couples who deal with children with life-threatening diseases end up in divorce. It was a stunning percentage and yet, at the same time, I believed it. Not that we were struggling, but just because big life events are hard, and people process things differently. It made us realize just how important the counseling was for us.

With everything going on, we had lots to talk about and each one-hour session went by quickly. We discussed Kendyl and her care, our relationship as a couple, career options for Zach, relationships with other family members, and more. We started going about once a month and continued for several months. These counseling sessions were really a blessing. Each one would have cost us about $100, and this was money that we didn't have. Some advice was deep, and some was simple but important, yet everything helped. Sometimes it's easier to receive advice from someone who isn't a family member. It's also helpful to hear an unbiased point of view from someone who isn't living the trial with you. I will be forever grateful for those counseling sessions and for the counselor who was so generous during our time of need.

The counseling was more helpful than anticipated. I realized that I was beginning to feel really low. My life seemed so depressing. I had gone through severe post-partum depression with my first baby and although it wasn't as severe this time, I could tell that I was struggling. I had experienced this feeling before and I didn't want it to get out of control again. The counselor helped me get in touch with a doctor who later helped me with depression and prescribed medication. I had worried about having to deal with post-partum depression after my second baby, but with the diagnosis, and everything else that was going on, it wasn't surprising. I'm not sure that I would have found this doctor without the counselor. He has continued to be my doctor for years.

Be aware of those who need help of any kind. You never know when you might be the one who connects those who can help with those in need.

September 2016

We were getting used to having Kendyl home and life in the post-transplant stage was under control. I knew that I needed to start taking care of myself again. It was hard to admit, but I was bigger at this point than right after my second pregnancy. I realized that the bad habits I had created needed to stop. Kendyl needed me, and I wanted to take care of her in the best way that I could. I realized that if I wanted to be around for her and have the energy to care for her like I wanted to, I needed to make myself a priority. I needed to take control again. For a while, I truly felt that I didn't have anything to look forward to except putting the girls to bed and having some ice cream or treats. That is embarrassing to admit, but it is the truth. I didn't do this every single night, but it happened more often than it should have.

I had been a runner for years and used to love it. I didn't enjoy training, but I loved running races (mostly half marathons) and thought I would do that for life. After having two kids and with a complicated med schedule to follow, it was really hard. My parents had even bought me a fancy double-Bob stroller, but it was challenging to take Kendyl and her feeding equipment along. I realized that I needed something new, which I could do from home.

I had watched my sister doing some programs at home and decided to look into it. One day, while my mom was doing her makeup in her bathroom, I began talking to her about trying out this fitness thing and the idea of joining this community. I didn't bring it up to Zach because I didn't want to stress him out. I was feeling bad for him that he still didn't have a job, despite all his efforts. My mom told me that I might as well try.

I decided to go for it and signed up a week later, while in the hospital again (spoiler alert), and fell in love with it! I loved that I could get a good workout from my home while right next to the girls. It was amazing that I could take care of them and me at the same time. I also enjoyed not worrying about germs. I felt strongly that I wanted to stay accountable and inspire others and knew this would keep me focused on my journey too.

Now, let me be clear about one thing. We all go through seasons. There are seasons when it just might not be possible to exercise and, in my opinion, it is OK if it's temporary. But I knew Kendyl's care was going to be long-term, and I needed to change. While being in the hospital, it felt like the only thing exciting in my life was visitors or going downstairs to get something to eat.

It seemed like the worst timing ever to start something new, but I couldn't get rid of the feeling in my heart that I needed to do this. While it might appear to be something drastic, it felt like it would be good for me. Looking back now, I know it was the perfect time for me to start my journey as it still continues today.

Listen to those tugs in your heart.

September 11, 2016

Kendyl had now been home from the hospital for two and a half weeks. She woke up this morning and her eye was puffy, swollen and almost closed shut. It got worse throughout the day. She later started having a fever, so my mom and I took her to the ER around 9 p.m. that night. There is no good time to go, but nighttime is the worst, in my opinion, because you are tired, and it takes hours to be seen. I can't remember the details but for some reason I was mad at Zach. We got in a small fight before I left, nothing big but I was frustrated. He hadn't done anything wrong, but stress and depression can do weird things sometimes. For whatever reason, I didn't want him to go with me and I was a brat to him as we left home.

Kendyl was finally seen by doctors and moved to an inpatient room after midnight. I was so tired and drained, physically, and emotionally. We were told that she had an eye infection. Her little body and immune system were so suppressed, in order to not reject her new organ, that she had developed this infection just from scratching her eye.

It really is amazing what happens when you don't have an immune system. Little things like this are often taken for granted. It was hard to see her little eye so red and swollen, but we were thankful that it wasn't her liver that had brought her back in; it was doing well.

I didn't mean to be a brat that night. I truly wasn't frustrated with Zach, but I took it out on him, and it wasn't fair. I now try to remember this if words or actions hurt my feelings. We never know what people are going through.

In stressful situations, many people are on the verge of breaking down. It is quite easy to do things that might hurt their feelings without even realizing.

September 14, 2016

My parents and my sister came to visit us. We were told there was dinner and a party going on in the Ronald McDonald Room. Different people would often bring in dinners for those staying in the hospital. I usually didn't go, but this night they said they were having a party. It sounded a little fun to try something new, so I went with my mom and dad while my sister stayed back in the room with Kendyl.

As we approached the room, we noticed a sign on the door about a birthday party for a little boy who would have been turning one year old that day. This boy only lived 10 hours, despite having had five surgeries while in utero.

Dinner and cake were provided and as we were leaving, they offered presents for kids. They had gifts wrapped by age range and gender. They gave us a gift not only for Kendyl, but one for Alyx as well. I was so touched by their generosity.

My heart hurt for this angel mother and her family. I was impressed by her generosity as she was thinking of others on a sad day. While we talked to her, she shed a few tears and was so very sweet. She asked why we were there and a little bit about Kendyl's story. I admired this family for honoring their son by doing something for other families who had children admitted in the hospital. What an amazing family! I will always be grateful that we went to get dinner that night and experienced this.

When you are hurting, you often don't feel like serving (at least I don't). But serving others around you helps not only you, but the people you serve. The quickest way for us to feel better when we are sad is to serve others. I hope to never forget this example shown that day. This sweet mom had every reason to stay home in her pajamas and eat chocolate by herself, but instead she was helping others in their time of need. Even though she cried a little as we talked to her, it was inspiring to see her smile too. This birthday party and experience changed my mood about everything as I realized just how blessed and lucky I was. I could have it far worse than I really did.

September 20, 2016

Kendyl came home once again. It was great to be back home and to have my girls together again. To this day, there is a still a small scar off to the side of her nose by her eye. It is a reminder of just how fragile she was.

October 1, 2016

We finally celebrated our little miracle girl's first birthday. Alyx had been sick, so we had postponed it. We had a little party, and we all wore our Kendyl Strong shirts. We had a cute cake that was shaped like a onesie, and we had pictures of Kendyl around the room. At the party, I also went through her short but eventful life with a journal where I had written down each hospital stay. She had spent a total of 111 days during her first year of life. It had no doubt been a hard year, but there were many blessings.

This is something I had recorded in my journal about the blessings:

Kendyl didn't live in the hospital waiting for a liver (several kids do). She was very sick but never in the critical 1A/1B status. She was able to fly to Utah before she got too sick. We have an amazing liver team at Primary's and especially her doctor. Kendyl was home and not in the hospital the weekend in May when I got to see my grandma and other family that I didn't see often. Most of all, she is alive today because of a new liver and donor family and she is doing awesome!

October 8, 2016

It was a beautiful day celebrating my grandma who had passed away. It was sad for me and my family, yet we were happy that she could rest in peace. Seeing her in the casket at the viewing, my heart was hurting as the last time I had seen her was in May. Although we lived very close, we did not visit her often because she was in a seniors' residence, and I worried about catching germs and bringing them home. From the time I saw her in May until today, Kendyl had been very fragile. Even before the transplant, as we waited on a liver, we worried about catching something that could cause her to not be eligible for surgery. After the transplant, I knew I had to remain cautious due to her anti-rejection meds being so high to help avoid organ rejection.

Parents make sacrifices for their kids all the time. When you have a child that has certain needs, I believe the sacrifices increase. I've often pondered about this experience and wondered if I would have done anything differently if I had known what would happen. Honestly, I believe I did the right thing, although I wish I could have seen my grandma again before she passed. I strongly believe that once she passed, she knew my situation and understood my decision. I believe that she felt that I did the right thing too.

The memories that I have of my grandma are pure treasures for me. When Zach and I got married, we lived next door to her and tried to help her out whenever we could. We would invite her for dinner, take her garbage out, and take her to church with us. Those are fond memories that I hold dear to my heart. I didn't see my grandma at the end when she was very sick, but I believe I had the best time with her during those years before her health started declining.

October 11, 2016

Although it was difficult, I felt strongly about writing a letter to Kendyl's donor family. It was something we immediately started working on once she came home from the hospital. It did feel like an overwhelming task. I don't consider myself to be a writer (funny that I wrote this book) but it also felt silly to write a thank you message for saving our daughter's life. It was hard to know what to say, or how to say it, which is probably why most people are intimidated to write. I knew in my heart that even though it was hard, I could never adequately share how grateful I was. I tried as best as possible to express our gratitude and sent it along with a few pictures of Kendyl. When I read it now, there are things that I would like to change, but this is what was sent. I share this to maybe help or inspire someone else who might be considering writing something similar. I know it isn't perfect by any means, but I share in case it can help someone.

Dear Family,

We are sure this letter may be bittersweet to read. It is both painful and joyous. It is difficult for us to write and express the feelings that we have. We have wanted to send this letter since the day of our daughter's transplant but have found it difficult to express all of our feelings. We wanted to do our best to try and thank you for the gift of your child's liver that you have given to our family.

We can't imagine what you are going through and what it would be like to lose a child. We hope this letter will bring you some peace. We can't imagine what it was like to try to make that decision in such a time when your hearts were broken and devastated. We will forever be grateful for your decision.

Because of you and your precious child, our child is alive today. Our daughter was born with a genetic problem called Biliary Atresia. We received the diagnosis when she was 2 months old. A week later she had major surgery to help her liver function properly. We were devastated a few weeks later when we learned that the surgery was unsuccessful, and she would need a liver transplant in the near future. Our daughter was put on a waiting list, and we watched her get sicker every day. A long four months later we received the news that your precious family had decided to give us the gift of life. We will never forget the day we put our little girl of only 9 months into the surgeon's hands to perform one of the largest operations. We have an amazing doctor, surgeon, and team but they were not the ones to save her life. It was you. Although we knew nothing about where the liver was coming from, what the gender of the baby was, how old the baby was, etc. we felt immediate and indescribable love for this baby and family.

We want you to know that we are diligent about taking care of our daughter because we love her but also because if we didn't, we would feel as though the precious liver was wasted. The care that our daughter requires is not easy, but we are very grateful she is alive.

Our little girl has an older sister who adores her. It has been that way since the day she was born. They are best friends and have a special bond. As we watched our baby get sicker and realized that without a new liver, she wouldn't live much longer, our thoughts always went to our oldest child. We wondered how we would give her that news if she was to lose her sister. Thinking of losing either one of our girls breaks our hearts but thinking of explaining it to the other one breaks our hearts even more. We hope that if your sweet child has a sibling(s) they will know that we think of them often as well.

Our little girl has always had a sweet spirit about her. She has been through a lot in her lifetime and yet is always smiling and happy. Although she is little for her age, she melts everyone's hearts with her large amount of hair and big personality. She absolutely loves her sister and smiles more for her than anyone else. She loves to be held, tickled, read to, and she especially loves her binky. She is now getting close to crawling and standing. She still has a feeding tube and is slowly learning to eat by mouth. (Because she has been sick for so long, she has been tube dependent most of her life.) She is the light in our lives and many others.

Having a new liver has completely changed her life. She is doing well, and we are very grateful. We look forward to her growing up and being able to be a normal kid. We are beyond grateful we will be able to see what she will do with her life and look forward to her having her own family someday.

Your selfless sacrifice and kindness mean that our child has a bright future ahead of her. We think of you every single day and always will. We are still in awe that our baby has a liver from another precious child. We find ourselves often looking at our daughter and imagining what your sweet baby was like and what the amazing parents that made that decision are like. If there are any other details or information about our family or our little girl that you would like to know, we would be willing to share any information you would like. We think of you every day and you are always in our prayers.

Much Love,
Your Recipient Family

This is what was in our hearts when we sent it. We don't know that family, but we know they have accepted the letter (the family had the option to receive it or not). We still hope to hear back from them one day, but we know that our chances are slim at this point. Even though we might never meet them, they remain in our thoughts, and we are forever grateful for their selfless gift of life.

Your words might not be perfect, but it's always worth trying to share your message as best as you can.

Fall 2016

One day I was feeling overwhelmed and angry with life. Not only were we dealing with Kendyl and her care but also with moving forward with our personal life. When Zach finished law school, he immediately started studying for his Bar Exam. After taking the test, he started looking for jobs. He would leave every morning for my parent's office. He treated it as a full-time job. He got a few interviews, and a few went so well that he felt confident that he would get the job. Some prospective employers even showed him where his desk would be. It was devastating to find out days later that he didn't get the job. It was really hard having him gone all day but not be bringing in any income. My heart broke for him as I knew he wanted to provide for his family and was working hard, but no jobs came.

I tried my best to be patient and lift him up, even though I was anxious for our own place. Zach is really good at handling stress, but I could tell it was really hard on him. It was heartbreaking to watch as he had worked so hard in school and yet it seemed like we still couldn't move forward. We went through mixed emotions when my dad found a job that he loved. We were sincerely happy for him, but it also stung a little, especially when we lived in the same house.

Life felt so unfair, and I was angry. I was driving by myself in the neighborhood one day when I started crying and yelling at God that I was mad at Him. I complained that this was too much to carry, and it wasn't fair. I could handle some of the situation but not all of it. Yet, I also promised that I would stay faithful and keep doing what I knew I should. Even though I was mad and told God that it seemed ridiculous, I wanted Him to know how I felt (even though I knew He already did).

I've heard it said that it's OK to be mad at God as long as you tell Him. I'm not sure that's true, but I do believe it's more productive to tell Him, rather than other people, how you feel about your frustrations. I feel that simple experience strengthened my relationship with God. It is OK to be mad at God, but I believe He wants to hear about our lives and that He wants to hear it from us.

November 7, 2016

Kendyl was doing fine in the morning, but things changed quickly. She started not feeling well and we were worried it was dehydration, so we decided to take her to the ER. This can be a serious issue for transplant kiddos, so we quickly made arrangements for Alyx and packed up to take Kendyl in.

Because she had been throwing up, I wanted to ride next to her in the back for the hour-long car ride to the hospital. With all the luggage and supplies for her stay, and not enough room for me to sit, we moved Alyx's empty car seat to the front passenger seat. At this point we didn't know how long we would be there and wanted to keep it in the car, so that was the easiest place to put it.

We waited in the ER for several hours until we finally got settled into a room at 1 a.m. When Zach went out to get our luggage from the car, he found a note on the windshield that read, "Hey, lesson of the day. Kids under the age of 12 or in a car seat are meant to be in the backseat.—17-year-old mom who follows the law."

We found it frustrating that someone would take the time to write this when they clearly had no idea what our situation was. It was annoying to see the note at a time when we were tired, worried, and had been trying to do our best for our little girl. I would like to think that if this person knew our situation, they would understand and have compassion. But they didn't know and chose to leave the note. This was a powerful lesson for me. Luckily, this stay was for nothing major, just a little virus that affected her immune-suppressed body harder than it would for others. Luckily, Kendyl came home the next day.

You truly never know someone's situation or
their struggles. Be kind and don't judge.

November 14, 2016

We had an appointment at home with someone from Early Intervention, a program to enhance growth and development in babies or toddlers with developmental delays or disabilities. The therapist visiting hadn't seen Kendyl since June, just before the transplant, when she was very sick. At that time, she couldn't move by herself at all and wouldn't eat anything by mouth. She couldn't even spend time on her tummy because her belly was so big that it caused pain. Her skin tone was also very yellow. The therapist was amazed to see how far she had come. Today she saw a very different little girl who was moving around, sitting by herself again (had to relearn after transplant) and was close to walking.

As the months went on, Kendyl gradually got rid of some meds. We celebrated each one that was eliminated from her schedule. Not only was it exciting to know that her body didn't need a certain medicine anymore, but it was also relieving that we had one less to worry about. It felt like a full-time job trying to get all her meds refilled at different times and picking them up. It was a lot to balance. I would joke all the time that I needed a secretary just to keep track of her meds and doctor appointments. Wouldn't it be nice if we all had a secretary for our lives?

Life was still challenging. It was hard not being able to take her anywhere because of germs and her suppressed immune system. It was difficult to stay home a lot and painful to not be able to take my older daughter out or to attend church as a family.

November 18, 2016

I had the opportunity to give blood. I had done it a few times before, but this time it was more meaningful to me. Kendyl had already had a few blood transfusions and would most likely have several more in the future. Liver transplants use the most blood of any organ transplants. Because Kendyl received a liver from a donor with a different blood type, each time she needs blood she requires a special kind that is "washed."

Blood is always needed, not only for transfusions, but for transplants and accidents as well. There are many safety rules for giving blood. Unfortunately, many people can't donate because of health conditions or lifestyle. In my area, I particularly like to support ARUP Blood Services because they provide the blood for Primary Children's Hospital.

If you can give blood, please do it. This is a simple way to burn up to 650 calories, and more importantly, you can save others' lives.

November 19, 2016

Big news in our house! There was a new walker. I got the cutest video of Kendyl walking with her little walker and it just about melted my heart. I'm not sure who was prouder, me or her. Every milestone for little ones is exciting, but there is something even more special when they have been through so much.

Zach's sister made us laugh when she said that Kendyl learned to walk faster than her daughter did, yet she had spent half her life in a hospital bed.

November 23, 2016

Kendyl pulled her tube out again and was able to be tube-free most of the day. I wanted to give her face a break from all the tape and see how she would do drinking water by mouth throughout the day. Our goal was 120 milliliters (4 ounces), but she drank even more than that. This doesn't seem like much, but for Kendyl it was huge.

It was a great day watching her eat, walk and crawl without the annoying tube holding her back. It was sad putting a new one back in before bedtime, but it made us smile to see some amazing progress. I was feeling very grateful.

Don't compare your journey.
Focus on your own progress.

November 24, 2016

It was Thanksgiving Day and Kendyl was doing well. We celebrated with family at a hotel in Salt Lake. It was nice enjoying all the holiday food without having to cook. We had a great time with our family, and we all celebrated having Kendyl with us. It was the first time that we used the highchair cover that we had for Alyx to protect her from germs. She was over a year old, so this simple observation showed that we didn't take her out much. We spent the night at the hotel and the next morning I drove to the hospital (which was close to the hotel). Even on a holiday week, our girl still needed labs. She was doing well but she still had to be checked regularly; still needed her feeds, her meds, etc.

November/December 2016

The doorbell rang. Since it wasn't my house, I rarely got the door, but I was close and decided to answer. There was no one on the porch but I found an envelope addressed to Zach and Sami. As I opened it up and felt how thick the envelope was, I couldn't even speak. I counted the money and it seemed as if there was no end in sight. This is a moment I'll never forget. It meant so much to me that people would be this generous and it touched my heart to know that someone was thinking of us. A few days later, we had a very similar experience. I was shocked and very grateful. I still wish I knew who was so generous to us and thank them for making a difference in our lives.

This act of kindness left a mark on our hearts and inspired us to anonymously give for Christmas each year. The amount isn't close to what we received that night, but we do try to think of others and give what we can.

December 7, 2016

Because Kendyl was in the Early Intervention program, we benefited from special opportunities. One of them was having Santa visit our house. The girls loved it! It was fun to get pictures with him and enjoy the magic of the holiday.

Although Kendyl was little, I mostly appreciated it for Alyx as she went through a lot too and frequently missed out on things because of her sister. We didn't dwell on it but as parents it was easy to notice and feel bad for Alyx. Seeing Santa was just not a realistic option for us at the time. Having a sick child opened my eyes to so many amazing organizations and companies that help families in challenging situations like ours.

December 13, 2016

It felt like we were on vacation. It was the first week Kendyl didn't have labs since her transplant that was in July! This was a big deal for her, and we were grateful. We felt blessed that she was doing well and even graduated from physical therapy because she was right back on track for her age.

December 20, 2016

They say that "third times' the charm," right? Zach had another interview for the same company which had hinted about hiring him. He was skeptical to interview again as he had never heard anything back from them. However, this time he was offered the position. Not only did he get a job that he liked, but the location was also better. He still works there today and absolutely loves it. Having the other two positions fall through turned out to be a blessing, so it was well worth the wait.

December 25, 2016

Merry Christmas! It was a crazy Christmas as we were still living at my parents, but it was a wonderful day. I think it was fun for my parents to be able to see the magic of Christmas morning through our little ones. It was a happy day. We didn't have our own place, but it was much better than being in the hospital, like the year before, and having Kendyl doing so well was the best gift we could have asked for. We felt truly blessed and grateful.

December 26, 2016

It was the day after Christmas, but it felt like the real holiday and was the highlight of our Christmas. We broke the rules and took Kendyl to church with us. She hadn't been to church since May. All I wanted was to spend Christmas together (not in the hospital) and when I found cute and cheap matching red sweater dresses for the girls, I decided to take her with us. It was so wonderful to be there. This was the best Christmas day and present for our family.

Life is about outfits. (Just kidding.) But really, matching outfits for my girls make me really happy. I still appreciate the pictures that I took that day. I am fairly confident that they don't remember that day or their dresses, but I do. I know that the money I spent for that day was well worth it for me.

Even if money is tight, it's OK to do something that makes you happy. It's often the little things that bring the most joy.

December 28, 2016

We saw a townhome that was for rent not too far from our parents' house and decided to go see it. We loaded up the kids in the car and drove by. It looked nice from the outside so we called to see if we could make an appointment to see inside. On the way home, both girls fell asleep. This was a rare occurrence on such a short drive. With both girls comfortably sleeping, we decided to drive around and see if there were any other homes we wanted to look at. We saw a few and then we stumbled upon a home in a cute neighborhood that we were interested in. It was easy to see that no one lived there, so we called and booked a visit later that day.

As we walked through the house, we immediately knew it could be a wonderful home for our family. Many improvements had been made which made it even more enticing. We wanted to have our parents see it too, so they came the next day for a walkthrough. After the visit, we told the owner that we would get back to him soon, but he informed us that he would be showing it to someone else later that day. I didn't know it at the time, but after the visit with our family, my father-in-law told the owner, "Cancel your next appointment. We want it." We later called and told him that we wanted to rent the home. We were so excited!

About six months before we even started looking for a place, I had this vivid thought that we would end up in that neighborhood. I immediately dismissed it and thought, "There's no way." We had lived with family for so long that I was ready to live a good distance away. However, this home turned out to be the perfect one for us.

December 30, 2016

We legally signed the papers that made us official renters! Zach had not even started working yet but he was going to begin his new job at the start of the new year. Money was tight so we asked if there was any way to hold the home for a month as moving in for February would be better for us. The owner told us that he wouldn't normally do that, but for us he was willing to do it. I often look back on the experience and think about how trusting he must have been to sign a contract when we didn't even have a job yet, and then holding the home for us for a month. I'm not sure I would have trusted us like this, but I'm forever grateful he did. I couldn't wait to have our own home again. It had been a year and I was so ready. I was looking forward to getting our things out of storage. It felt like it had been forever.

December 31, 2016

I was happy and excited to see 2016 come to an end. It was quite a year. I will never forget that year and would never wish a similar one, filled with so many heartaches, to anyone. Even though it was the hardest year of our lives, it also brought many blessings and shaped us into the people we are today. It helped me recognize just how good life can be. I since appreciate the good times ahead of us instead of taking them for granted. It made us stronger and taught us lessons that we would never have learned any other way.

2016 was a hard year for us and we could dwell on that, but I have chosen to focus on all the good from that year. My daughter received her gift of life, my dad was available to help us move home, my mom was able to fly home with my oldest daughter, and Zach finished school and was offered a job that he was excited for. These are just a few of the things I like to focus on and remember.

There are always two ways to look at things. You can look for the positive or you can look for the negative. Both positive and negative exist in every situation. What will you choose to focus on?

Chapter 3
LiveReal
2017

January 3, 2017

I t was an exciting day to have Zach begin his job at the bank. We had been through a lot, and it was nice to start the year with something so positive. It finally felt like we were getting on our feet again. Zach has always been a very positive guy. He doesn't easily stress, he is easy-going, and has a positive outlook on life. I loved that about him from the day I met him.

Of course, I was thrilled when he started his job, but most of all I was excited for him. As the rock of our family, I was happy for him that he could feel that he was providing for his family and that school had been worth it (for a minute we wondered).

Everyone shows their emotions differently. Zach doesn't talk or display his feelings often, but today I could see and feel it. I trusted that this day would come, and while I was anxiously waiting for it, I tried to be uplifting and patient throughout the journey. I believe it is important to look out for your spouse, especially in tough times, whether they seem fine or not.

Your spouse or other people around you might not always express their feelings, but deep down, they might be struggling more than you know.

January 25, 2017

Today I learned about another child that lost their battle to Biliary Atresia. The poor little girl didn't receive a liver in time. I don't know the child or her family, but my heart was broken for them. I couldn't imagine what they were going through.

As I watched my little Kendyl climb on a chair, get a blanket, and a storybook (all by herself of course), I could not help but feel so grateful and pleased with her progress. When I hear of other babies or kids that didn't make it, I can't help but wonder how we got so lucky. Why was I one of the lucky moms blessed to have my child survive? Why was it that the only way our baby could live was if another one did not? I still wonder why.

Yet, I am reminded that it is all in God's hands. I will admit that some days, Kendyl completely exhausted me. She was so active and explored everywhere. She was up and down the stairs, getting into places where she should not be, and it seemed as if she would not only be walking, but running by the next day! I was not always as patient with her as I should have been. I lost her binky (pacifier) several times and spent way too much time trying to find it. While looking for binkies and chasing her, I was also packing up our stuff to move. Packing with little ones is not easy or convenient. However, even on a tiring day, she reminded us that every day is a gift.

It is OK to feel tired. When we watch someone else go through a difficult time, we understand why they are tired and need a break.

Give the same grace to yourself
as you would to someone else.

February 2017

A toddler on a feeding tube is not a simple thing. They move around so fast while discovering their new independence. When it was time for Kendyl to have a feed, we often had to wear the backpack with the feeding tube and stay in her pursuit. It was a good workout. Sometimes we would even have Alyx wear the backpack and chase her. It was hilarious to watch them. You know those moments when you just have to laugh? This was one of them.

February 4, 2017

It was our official moving day. Our belongings had been stored since Zach brought it down after finishing school in May. It had been a whole year since I had access to most of my clothes. Looking back, I was grateful that I did not know it would be that long. When I packed up my stuff to come to Utah, I thought it would only be for a few months. I had no idea it would stretch to be an entire year.

We moved in with help from family and some of Zach's co-workers. We got somewhat settled while the girls played at a cousin's house. Because of all the help we had, we were able to get beds set up, toys out, and get mostly unpacked.

We later picked up the girls and brought them to our new home. They had seen it once before when it was empty, but it was exciting to show them their room and especially the toy room with all their dolls, stuffed animals, and toys. Zach and I watched with awe, their big smiles, and happy tears when they got reunited with their toys after a full year. It melted our hearts to see them with toys that had been forgotten and to finally be in our own space again. It was such a happy moment for our family.

I will be the first to admit I hate the word patience, but it really is important. I cannot say that this is my strongest skill or that I demonstrate it often enough, but I had to develop and use it frequently. Being forced to be patient allowed great things to come and I appreciated them so much more when they finally arrived.

When you have to wait for something, it often makes it so much sweeter. Learn to enjoy the anticipation.

February 6, 2017

I had been wanting to get a picture with the surgeon who did Kendyl's transplant since the day of her surgery, but I never had the chance. At a follow-up visit today at the hospital, we ran into Dr. K, and I was thrilled to finally get a picture with him.

February 17, 2017

I celebrated a bittersweet accomplishment today. I was able to put Kendyl's feeding tube in completely by myself. She pulled it out at least three times this week, so I had a lot of practice. I guess it's good news that I can now put it back in without help. If you find yourself in this situation or know someone who might be, here are my tips. Strap them in their infant car seat with the handle back so they are almost sitting up (it is easier if they are sitting up vs. lying down). Have your supplies ready and put them in front of the TV to distract them. It is not fun, but it will not last long. Go for it and good luck. Be sure to give them lots of snuggles after.

February 20, 2017

Kendyl had an IVIG Infusion (intravenous immune globulin) which is antibodies that can be given through a vein. They are proteins that your body makes to help fight infections. This was a safe way to boost her immune system. It took most of the day, but I was grateful we did not have to be admitted. As she stood in her crib jumping and trying to climb out, she kept saying her new favorite word over and over, "no, no, no."

February 2017

As we continued to get settled into our home, I was amazed by how much we had stored and how badly we needed to go through it. Most people would declutter and have a garage sale or give to charity before moving. We did not have that option because it was such a quick decision for us to move.

While going through a random box, which was most likely the contents from a junk drawer from our Spokane house, I found a message from a fortune cookie. I laughed when I saw that this piece of paper had made it all the way from Washington to Utah. I also felt grateful for those who had packed up my home when I was not able to so. When I told my mother-in-law about this, she also laughed and told me she did not want to throw anything away because it was not hers. I appreciate that she did not try to go through my things but simply packed up everything in my home for me, including a simple fortune cookie message.

This was a reminder about how crazy our life had been and how much had happened. The fortune said, **"Your best investment is in yourself."** I still keep that message in my office to remind me to keep things in perspective when facing difficult situations. I thought that if a small fortune cookie message had made it this far, it must be important. And I still believe it is.

March 2017

I was grateful about an idea I had that was beyond me, an answer to prayer that I felt was from God. The idea had been to mix PediaSure with water. I had been told by the liver team to try it with different kinds of milk, but I knew that Kendyl did not really like milk-based food because she had regurgitated so much of it. I started with a mix that was mostly water and little PediaSure, but slowly inverted the ratio to use less water. It seemed to work pretty well and I considered it a brilliant idea.

If we listen and pay attention, God can help us with all things, both big and small.

March 10, 2017

Kendyl was feeling 'bigger' to me, meaning she was doing big kid things. I took her to the hospital to have some of her prescriptions filled and for an ultrasound. She had had us on our toes over the last few days since some of her labs looked a little off. Although they were not exactly sure why, her doctors were not too worried because the labs and ultrasound looked good from today. I felt so relieved. I was grateful for being close to my mom as she could help us get out the door and watch Alyx all day. It did not seem to matter how early I got up; I was always late heading out the door with everything I needed to prepare for a full day out with Kendyl.

March 15, 2017

Kendyl spent over 36 hours without a feeding tube! It had been great to let her have a bath in the big tub, scratch her nose without worrying that she might pull her tube out, and not add more bruises on her body from the tube. Her poor back had several large bruises from sleeping on the tube at night. Medications without the tube was stressful and I had to get a little creative. We had to do a lot of calculations to make sure she was getting the calories she needed. It was also hard to watch her closely to make sure she didn't drink too fast and throw up. Since she had been dependent on a feeding tube for so long, we had to frequently check her glucose level as she wasn't being fed at night anymore. We had to poke her at both 2 a.m. and at 7:30 a.m. to make sure her blood sugar was stable. This was quite a challenge but worth it to watch her be tube-free for that long.

March 19, 2017

After Kendyl's last liver appointment, we were given the OK to start taking her out a little bit. There was a special Ward Conference meeting at our church and Zach and I both wanted to hear our leaders. It was wonderful to be there as a family again. We thought Kendyl would sleep for most of it, but that didn't happen! It made me smile to watch her look at everything around us with curiosity. She really did not like staying in such a little space on the bench, but we made it through. It was also a proud moment to hear Alyx give her second talk in Primary. She did great! My heart was full. God is good!

March 25, 2017

We celebrated Kendyl being 18 months old by having early morning labs. What a journey. She was the cutest, sweetest, and busiest little bundle. I have always been so honored to be her mom. It was a year ago on this day that she had been listed on the transplant list. I was grateful this was now behind us. She was doing well for the most part except for a condition called Clostridium difficile Colitis, or known as C. diff, which causes severe diarrhea and colitis. She was also dealing with a few other complications, but we were so proud of her strength and attitude through it all. She had been through so much in her short life, yet she carried on as if everything was just normal.

March 27, 2017

People are so thoughtful and kind. I opened the door today to a sweet neighbor holding flowers. She told me she had been touched by the talk I had given in church the previous day. I was amazed and felt I truly did not deserve them, but I was touched by her gesture. This sweet woman brightened up my day and inspired me to follow her thoughtful example whenever I could. You can never go wrong with flowers; they are always appreciated.

April 3, 2017

My mom and I took Kendyl to her early labs together and while at the hospital, decided to donate blood. We tried to give as often as possible because we knew how important blood transfusions had been to save Kendyl's life. It felt like a simple way to serve and give back.

I had a moment where I realized how much my life had changed over the past several months. My efforts in trying to take better care of myself were now becoming habits. Knowing that I would not be able to exercise for hours after giving blood, I had set my alarm for 4:30 a.m. that morning. This allowed me to read, do a workout, get to labs on time and donate blood. I was amazed of these accomplishments, especially after being up until midnight to give Kendyl a medication. I had felt stuck for so long, and I wanted to be different and feel better. It was working!

Acknowledge yourself. Important changes can happen gradually over time without even noticing.

April 10, 2017

It was another long day but both girls were so good. Kendyl had two pokes and a blowout. She still had a few minor complications but overall was doing well and most of her labs looked good. Our biggest concern was now her weight as she had lost over a pound since her last appointment. Her arms and legs were so tiny. She was growing taller but was several pounds behind where she should have been. While she was eating more every day, she was very picky.

It was entertaining to watch Kendyl during our appointment with her liver team. She was wearing little white socks, baby moccasins and a diaper. Her clothes were off so that they could weigh her. Because they watched her weight so closely, each time we entered the exam room we would change her into a clean diaper and that's the only thing she would keep on while being weighed. As always, we would discuss her labs and care routine with her doctor. While we talked, Kendyl would grab all of her meds and formula from our small insulated cooler bag. She would pull out one at a time, put them all on the floor, and then put them back in the cooler. My mom and I watched her do this several times during the visit. I was happy that something so simple could keep her occupied for so long.

April 12, 2017

Zach and his work team had a dinner, play, and overnight stay in a hotel. I had been looking forward to this exciting evening to have some time alone with Zach and meeting his co-workers and their spouses. Instead, Kendyl was admitted to the hospital following concerns about her throwing up and her recent weight check. The team felt she needed to be checked to evaluate what was going on. I really felt sad that we had missed out on our plans. However, I then realized that Kendyl had not been in since November and that was a huge milestone. It was amazing to realize she had been able to stay home all through the respiratory and flu season. It was a miracle that she went the whole winter without being hospitalized.

One of the hardest parts of being a parent of a child with health issues is that you miss out on a lot. It's always disappointing to miss out on things, but I will say that over time it does get a bit easier.

April 14, 2017

Kendyl and I were sleeping peacefully in her hospital room when we were awakened at 6:30 a.m. They told us that we had to gather our things and move to a different room since ours was needed for a cancer patient. It was super annoying, but I totally understood the situation. It broke my heart to see and hear of more kids being diagnosed with cancer.

While I had been so excited about Kendyl drinking more, it was short-lived. She wasn't tolerating the PediaSure anymore, so we needed to make a change. My baby had been through a lot over the past few days. She had been poked for labs, had a biopsy done on her skin to look at a rash, and had a new feeding tube placed in her nose. We were impressed how she handled it like a champ. Most of the time she would go through it and not even cry. The nurses kept mentioning how tough she was; little but fierce. Although the results from the allergy test were clear, there was an issue with this formula. Since she had been struggling to keep her weight up, we could not spend more time trying to figure it out. We needed to make a change and found a new formula called EleCare Jr. This one seemed to sit better in her stomach and was easy for her little body to digest. We were grateful that the insurance would cover this as it was going cost about $1,800/month. We would now focus on her gaining weight again.

May 15, 2017

We were thrilled as Kendyl had a liver clinic doctor appointment, and she did not need to have labs again for an entire month. Her doctor said she was looking great, and everything was well with her liver. It was another tiring and busy Monday but so reassuring to hear this. We were still working on her weight by feeding the new high-calorie formula while also trying to get her to eat regular food. I never thought that a month off from labs would be a reason to celebrate, but it definitely was.

May 29, 2017

I woke up in a little bit of a funk. We were going swimming at my in-laws, but I was feeling sad that Kendyl would not be joining us because of her feeding tube. After living without one for a little bit, it was hard to have it back in. I had been looking forward to finally watch both my girls swim together.

Zach quickly reminded me that last year, on Memorial Day, we were worried about visiting her grave someday. We did not know if she would get a liver in time and tried to prepare ourselves in case the worst were to happen. After this reminder, the tube didn't seem so bad. I was beyond grateful that she was with us. I am so appreciative for my husband's positive attitude.

Perception really changes everything.

June 11, 2017

Kendyl went to the church nursery for the first time today. This was a big milestone for her. Most kids start attending when they are around 18 months old, but we had been nervous about germs, so we kept her away until now. She only went for the second hour and participated by singing, listening to a short lesson, coloring a picture, playing with bubbles, and watching the other kiddos eat a snack. We skipped the first hour as they play with toys, which is not a good thing for immune suppressed kiddos. I stayed with her and tried to give her a marshmallow while the kids were eating, but she gagged. She was not quite sure what to think of the other kids and they were not sure what to think of her. They kept pointing and looking at her feeding tube, which is a normal reaction.

I was touched by the nursery leaders who were happy to have her there and very understanding of her situation. They even sent some little toys home that matched the toys used when they sang different songs. I could wash and sanitize them so she would have her own set in the future.

June 12, 2017

We were approaching the one-year mark of Kendyl's transplant and were excited since we had heard many times, "Once you get through the first year after a transplant, everything will get better." Although she was doing well overall, it felt like her story was going to be different than what we had been told to expect.

We were happy with her progress of eating more by mouth, such as rice kernels (it is funny what you can get excited about!) At today's appointment with her liver team, they mentioned that Kendyl's portal vein, which had clotted soon after transplant, was now causing problems. They had not been worried about it earlier, but it was now a bigger problem and they felt like something needed to be done about it.

This is when we heard of Dr. R. again, the surgeon we had met a year prior, right after the transplant. We had been lucky to meet him before he joined the team. We were now looking at another surgery to fix the clotted portal vein. I thought it was fortunate that we had met this surgeon a year before moving here. It felt comforting that we knew and already trusted him. I do not believe in coincidences. I truly believe that the timing of meeting him after the transplant was meant to be. I know this was truly a tender mercy.

We often don't know the details of how
things come together, but God does.

June 15, 2017

It was another long day and most of it was spent at the hospital since Kendyl had a CT scan. It was supposed to only take two hours, but it took a lot longer. She had an IV placed for sedation. I'm not sure I will ever get used to seeing her be poked, but it all went well. She had CT scans before, so it was not a new experience, but she was way more active and verbal than before and it made me nervous. Watching her come out of anesthesia was funny. She was talking silly and wanted to walk in her crib. I could not seem to explain to her that it was not the best idea as the medication still in her system affected her balance.

The doctors had scheduled a procedure to place an NJ tube. (This tube is similar to the NG tube she currently had, but goes further down into the stomach, and it is placed in radiology to make sure it is in the right spot.)

Kendyl's weight had not increased at all since her last clinic appointment. However, for whatever reason (I had come up with a few in my mind), she stopped throwing up completely when we increased her feeds by mouth and through the tube. It seemed backwards to increase feeds and throw up less, but for whatever reason, she was doing much better and also seemed to be interested in eating solids again too. The new formula was making a difference.

I debated for a day or two but then decided that I was not going to put the tube in if it was not needed. Her doctor felt strongly that the NJ tube should be placed, and I totally understood why, but I told her that I wanted to wait. The team agreed to give Kendyl a one-week grace period but that was all. When we got checked in for the CT scan, I couldn't believe it when the scale said she had almost gained a pound in only a few days.

July 10, 2017

Kendyl did not look or act sick but her recent labs for the last few weeks had been elevated. They were not sure what was going on, so they wanted a liver biopsy. There was a chance that she might be going into rejection. It sounds scary, and it can be, but it isn't quite as bad as it appears to be. We were anxious for the results and knew it would be a long 24 hours waiting to hear back.

Even though our nerves were on the edge, I felt grateful that Kendyl seemed to be feeling good. I was relieved that Zach was able to come with me while family watched after Alyx. There were many unknowns and questions, but we continued to hope for some simple answers. Maybe it would be a simple virus or something like that. We prayed that it would not be a long hospital visit.

You never know what the future holds, but
you should hope for the best.

119

July 11, 2017

After a long day, we finally got some much-needed rest. Kendyl fell asleep in her stroller while we were on a little walk. She seemed peaceful so I brought her back to her room and she slept all night (except for when they came to check her vitals). During her biopsy, the previous day, she started bleeding internally and was admitted immediately, which turned out to be a blessing. We were initially going to be in the Rapid Transplant Unit for 24 hours but being admitted meant that she would be watched a little more closely. It also meant that I would have a couch bed instead of a chair to sleep in overnight. I had been up since 3 a.m. the previous day, so we were both worn out after such a long day.

The ultrasound showed that the bleeding had stopped, and we got the results of the biopsy which confirmed more good news. There was no rejection! However, there was the blood flow issue in her portal vein, so she would have a special ultrasound the following month to get a closer look. We were grateful that the biopsy was clear of rejection, and I was touched by all the text messages and love that we received from people who worried about her.

July 16, 2017

Before our immersion in the "transplant world," we had never heard the term "Liverversary." We quickly learned and realized how special these celebrations were and wanted to have one for our miracle girl. Our family all came together wearing our "Kendyl Strong" shirts. I hung up pictures of her journey and she opened a few gifts. My mom had even made a darling cake in the shape of a liver. I still remember how cute (and delicious!) it was with white frosting and green little dots around the edges. It was a wonderful day to look back on how far she had come.

Kendyl did not understand what we were celebrating, but we did. It was a little bittersweet to know she was doing well but also that another major surgery was on the horizon. Still, we enjoyed the day celebrating her gift of life. I love a quote that says, "Celebrate every tiny victory." Don't pass up moments to celebrate.

Celebrate anything that means something to you.

July 22, 2017

I had a lot on my mind. "Hurricane Kendyl," as we called her, was into everything. She had decided to refuse naps at the young age of 22 months old, and she no longer wanted to drink her formula by mouth. Since we were already in discussion of another surgery being possible, I wondered if it made sense for Kendyl to have a more permanent solution for her feeding needs. This was something that I had been pondering on a little bit. I knew nothing about this but kept feeling it might be a good option.

At the same time, she was still growing and melting our hearts in many ways, such as saying prayers. She was so smart and observant that she learned them on her own after watching her older sister. Even though I did not totally understand what she was saying, it was still the cutest thing. Witnessing her learning her prayers was the perfect reminder that I was the one who needed to pray.

July 30, 2017

We had a family homecoming at church at 9 a.m. It definitely was not easy to get there early with the medication schedule, but we did it. Being together at the meeting as a family was wonderful. I was not too surprised when I found myself out in the hall with Kendyl. She was restless and loud; not used to sitting still or being quiet.

I do not remember the details, but there was another parent in the hall with his son. I mentioned that my daughter was not used to sitting still in church and he replied that his son wasn't either. He then added that his son had a G-tube. I was so surprised by the coincidence since this had been on my mind a lot recently. When he asked if I wanted to see what it looked like, I immediately agreed. It was comforting to see that the little boy appeared to be thriving. I would have never guessed that he had a feeding tube and I hoped it would be the same for Kendyl.

What are the odds of this experience happening? The fact that we would attend that specific church meeting, where Kendyl would get fussy and that we would both be the only two parents in that hall at the same time, with kids, about the same age, dealing with similar issues. I believe this was an answer to my prayers. It was a sweet assurance that God was aware of my exact situation, and that He knew my concerns.

August 3, 2017

I would be lying if I said that my mind never went back to the past. Back to the time before learning that Kendyl had any health challenges. This was a day of ugly tears, from a heavy heart, with feelings that life was unfair, and fears that it would always be this way.

Kendyl had been giving me a really hard time lately. Almost two years old now, she was quite energetic and never held still as she was catching up on exploring everything. As an added challenge, she was continually throwing up and making a mess everywhere and was back to being completely dependent on her feeding tube. She required 10 medications in the morning and 8 every night, no matter what. To make things worse, Kendyl had a bad fall after climbing on our bed by herself. She had fallen onto the foot of the bed and hurt her cheek. Because she was taking aspirin, a blood thinner, she bled easily. On top of everything else, I now felt guilty that I didn't do enough to protect my fragile girl.

Accidents happen with kids whether they
have health issues or not. Do not feel guilty.

August 8, 2017

At today's liver clinic appointment, we were thrilled to see Kendyl's weight at 9 kilos, which I immediately calculated to be 21.5 lbs. However, the moment the doctor felt her tummy, she responded that the spleens were enlarged. This meant that she would not only need the blood routing surgery, but that she needed it a little sooner than expected. We had known that it was probably going to happen but wanted to make sure it was necessary because of the risks involved. The surgery known as Rex Bypass was scheduled that day for Thursday, September 28th.

There were multiple options for the surgery. The best option was to bypass the clot and bring the blood back into the liver. This would keep the liver healthy and happy so it would last longer. Another option was to bypass the clot by rerouting it a different way. We would not know which option would be the best until they got in there. We mentally prepared that the best-case option might not be possible, yet we hoped and prayed for the best.

Because of her slow progress in eating by mouth, we decided she would also receive a G-tube (gastrostomy tube) to replace her NG tube. It would be surgically placed in her stomach during the surgery, and we would access it on her tummy. This was an even more permanent solution than the NJ tube she had been scheduled to receive a few months earlier. We had hoped that she would learn to eat after the transplant and no longer need the tube. This is usually the case with most liver transplant kiddos, but it was not the case with Kendyl. It was a hard decision, but we felt at peace with it. She still struggled to eat and drink, and we knew that having a tube in her nose was not going to work long-term. As she was getting older and stronger, she would pull it out frequently. Putting it back was torturous for both of us as it was nearly impossible. I would have to hold her down (usually with someone else helping me) and put the tube up her nose (way farther than you would think) and it would then go down her throat and into her stomach. It was as traumatic as you would imagine. Not only was replacing the tube hard, but the tape that we used on her precious face to keep the tube in place was irritating her skin and leaving horrible rashes and redness. It hurt my heart to see how sore it was. We were also hopeful that with the tube out of her nose and throat she would want to eat more.

Because the G-tube was also being placed, there were two doctors and teams that had to coordinate the surgery. We were so grateful that they could do both procedures at the same time. Initially, my first reaction was feeling bad for her and myself as I was dreading another surgery with a long hospital stay. The minimum would be a two-week stay, but I knew it could be longer.

It was going to be a big surgery. The team told us that it could be longer than a transplant, which is typically eight hours, because it was such a detailed procedure. It was scary to think about her going through a major surgery again, but I held to the fact that Kendyl was much stronger now than before her transplant. She was bigger and her little body was ready. We hoped and prayed that all would go well and that this would be the answer to the prayer from a year earlier, that she would "heal quicker than anticipated" and it would be her last surgery for a long time.

August 21, 2017

We took Alyx to an amusement park near our house called Lagoon. To say it was a fun day was an understatement. It was fun to watch her smile and hear her giggle with so much excitement was worth every single penny. We had a blast with her while my mom watched Kendyl. We looked forward to the day when she would be able to join us too.

August 24, 2017

It was a good day, unlike most, which was welcomed. Our journey had taught us that things can change quickly, to be grateful for good days and not take them for granted. We played at the park, and I had a call with a friend from Spokane that I really missed.

I also attended the temple, which was quiet, peaceful, and beautiful. It had been way too long since I last attended. It was hard to get there as things seemed crazier than ever. Zach barely got home from work on time, Kendyl's feeding tube was loosely attached to her face, the girls were sad that I was leaving, and I knew time was short. I had mentioned that if the temple was too busy, I would come back home early to help with bedtime and medications. I thought to myself that if it was busy, God would know I had tried. When I arrived at the temple, I was surprised to see it was not busy and that I was able to get right in. It was a tender mercy moment for me. I left feeling humbled, uplifted, strengthened, loved, and had a greater determination to do my best.

August 26, 2017

We were able to watch Kendyl swim for the first time. It completely melted my heart and reminded me just how far she had come. Seeing her in her little swimsuit about killed me. She used to be so small and tiny! We had to be extra careful with her tube on her face, but it was worth it to see her rolls and thunder thighs. We were grateful that she was well enough to swim, yet I couldn't help but wonder what else was ahead.

I wrote this little part in my journal that day,

> *"She has pushed me to my limits (many times) and has made me wonder sometimes how I could possibly be the right mom for her. Although I fall short, I will always be grateful. Thank you Kendyl Rose, for teaching me about little moments and to not just have them pass by without enjoying them. Thank you for teaching me (or trying to teach me) to be happy no matter what you are facing. Thank you for your constant sweetness lately to give hugs and kisses and say prayers. I wish I could pause time right now. I am loving this stage. I love your sweet voice and all the words you say. For a little one who has spent*

a lot of her life in the hospital, you amaze me with how smart
you are. The fact that you still say Daddy every time I ask you
to say mommy shows you are smart and the little attitude you
have. I don't blame you for saying daddy. He is pretty great,
but you are welcome to say Mommy too. I cannot believe you
will be 2 years old next month. It's been quite the journey."

August 28, 2017

It was a big moment when I took both girls to the store and put Kendyl in the cart for the first time in her life. She was almost two years old, and it was a big deal to sit in the cart. While I did have a cart cover, I would usually keep her in her stroller to stay protected from germs. Because of the size of the stroller, I was only able to buy a few things at a time. It was nice today to have more room in my cart and be able to get more groceries. Alyx was also very excited about this. A new world had now been opened to us!

Although it was fun, I still preferred online shopping, especially for all the supplies we needed for Kendyl. Although she was such a little person, she got a lot of mail and packages, including baby wipes, diapers for during the day, thicker ones for the night, feeding supplies and more. What did we do before online shopping?

September 22, 2017

A family member bought a bracelet for me that said, *"Be stronger than the storm,"* it was sweet, and I absolutely loved it. I was feeling thankful for so many things. My heart really was full of appreciation for both little and big things, such as a random phone call, out of the blue, from someone wanting to help and give tips about G-tubes. But most of all, we loved receiving sweet words of encouragement, as many came right when we needed it. I often received messages exactly when I needed to know that I was doing the right thing and I had no doubt that these were not just coincidences. These little blessings showed me and reminded me that God is aware of us, and he loves us. Even when we fall short, when our hearts are heavy, and we feel we are not doing enough, He is there.

God helps us become stronger than the storm, whatever type of storm it may be.

September 25, 2017

My baby is now two years old! This miracle happened because of an organ donor. Most people say that time flies when their kids are growing up. Although I couldn't bring myself to say it had flown by, I really did not remember what life was like before Kendyl Rose joined our family. It had been quite the journey. Before she joined our family, I never once thought about my liver, spleen, feeding tubes, and lots of other things. I was amazed by everything I had learned in two years. Her life had brought a wide range of emotions in our lives. There were many difficult times, but it had absolutely been worth it. My little girl had taught me so much and continued to teach me daily. She taught me to be tough, to keep going, to laugh and most of all to love. Recently, she began giving the sweetest hugs and kisses, and I could not get enough of those.

We celebrated her birthday a day early because we were getting ready for her big surgery and Zach was busy at work to prepare to take time off. We also wanted to give her one more day to play with her new toys before going to the hospital. It was not a typical birthday, as it was a more spiritual celebration. Zach gave Kendyl and I beautiful blessings, and we fasted, and prayed as a family. We were at home as a family and that's all that really mattered. I felt grateful that she was little and did not expect much for her birthday. I could not believe that my baby had officially become a toddler.

The first few birthdays for kids are actually for parents and family because they do not really remember them. Keep that in mind if you are ever stressed about birthdays. Your kids will soon be old enough to tell you exactly what they want!

September 26, 2017

It was a very long day at the hospital. Kendyl had blood work, an ultrasound, and her final liver clinic visit before surgery. My nerves were on the edge, and I kept praying that all would go well while I was busy trying to prepare. Here I was cleaning the house, not knowing how long I would be gone. There was an inside joke between Zach and me that you could usually find me cleaning the tub on the day before a surgery. We laughed about it together, but I always felt better knowing that my home would be clean while I was gone and when we came back.

It can be a blessing to keep yourself busy,
especially during stressful times.

September 28, 2017

Just three days after her second birthday, Kendyl had her third major surgery, the Rex-Bypass. After trying to get a little bit of sleep, we arrived at the hospital at 5:45 a.m. It was scheduled at 7:30 a.m. for four and a half hours, but we were advised that it could potentially be longer.

After Kendyl was checked in and ready, the surgeon came to meet with us. He told us about the donor blood vessel that he was going to use and had us sign a form. Once again, all the feelings came back with the realization that our daughter was alive because of someone else, and we were being blessed once again through organ donation. We gave our final teary kisses a little before 8 a.m.

We waited in the same waiting room where we had been for the transplant. It was weird to be there again. In a way, it felt like we had just been there a few days earlier. As we waited there with our family, I was trying to process so many thoughts and emotions. I was sad and scared that my baby girl had to go through another surgery, but I was feeling grateful to have an amazing surgeon that we trusted performing the surgery. We waited for hours, and I kept thinking about the sweet snuggles I had gotten that morning while she was asleep. I was so grateful she had slept on me to pass the time, so she didn't notice if she was hungry. I was already looking forward to having more snuggles again. The team was really good at providing updates every hour. As we continued to wait, we kept trying to stay positive and to keep our minds occupied, we decided to see who could plank the longest between Zach and me. This was something I would have never imagined doing during a surgery, but I never pictured myself being the momma of a daughter who would have so many surgeries. (For the record, I won the plank contest.)

After several hours we decided to go to the cafeteria to get some lunch and hoped we could eat a little bit. I grabbed a salad and we all sat down at a table together as a family. We were not really saying much and noticed another large family eating nearby. Our focus turned to them, and it was easy to see that they had been crying. They had swollen and red eyes and my heart was hurting for them. A few minutes later they were crying again but also cheering a little bit. I wondered what had happened, what they had been through, and what their story was. Just like several other families I had seen in the hospital, I assumed that I would never know their story.

The surgery finally finished a little after 5 p.m. It took longer than expected but all went well. The surgeon was able to do the preferred option, which brought the blood back into her liver to be filtered. It was just as we had hoped as this normal way of routing is the best solution to keep the liver happy in the long-term. I was thrilled that they were able to do both the bypass and the G-tube at the same time. Although that was the plan, we knew there were going to be lots of risks and that they might not be able to accomplish both. After the surgery was completed, they moved us to a different waiting room. While we waited to see her, I noticed that two people from the large family in the cafeteria were there too. Shortly after, we were told we could see

Kendyl. The PICU had strict rules on visitors, so Zach stayed with his parents while I went with mine to see her. She was resting comfortably in the PICU and was already off the breathing machine. It was so great to see her, and she really looked good.

As Zach and his parents sat there, they noticed that the two persons in the waiting room had red eyes and looked sad. My father-in-law asked if they were OK. They opened up, through tears, to tell them about their precious granddaughter who had just passed away in a horse accident. They mentioned that they had received the news a few hours prior that she would be able to donate her organs. Zach and his parents thanked them for donating her organs and explained that Kendyl had a transplant last year.

Zach called me and told me to come back to the waiting room. He then introduced me and updated me on their story. My heart sank. I had remembered seeing the story on the news and their adorable little girl with big blue eyes and blonde hair who seemed to have such a sassy and funny personality from her pictures. My heart broke for them as they shared, through more tears, details of the story. We told them that we were thankful for their son and daughter-in-law's decision to have their little girl be an organ donor. They seemed to appreciate it and asked if we could meet the girl's parents. We all thought it might mean a lot to them, so we kindly agreed. Shortly after, we met them in the waiting room. They looked so sad and tired. We tried our best to express our thanks for their decision. We shared a little bit of Kendyl's liver transplant story and what it had done for our family. It was neat for us to be able to say thank you. There was not a dry eye in the room as we shared our experiences. Although it was not Kendyl's organ donor's family, it felt good to say thank you.

Over the following years, I have remained in touch with the Hale family. I am grateful for the opportunity to meet them and for the experience we shared.

Later, Zach and I spent a little more time with Kendyl. She was still sleeping and looked comfortable, so we said our goodbyes for the night and headed to a hotel close to the hospital. My generous and thoughtful parents had arranged that room so we could get some much-needed rest. It had been a big day and we were exhausted, physically and emotionally. Meeting that amazing family was such a special experience and there was such a sweet spirit as we spent time with them. I truly felt there was a reason that we met.

God puts people in our path so we can lift each other.

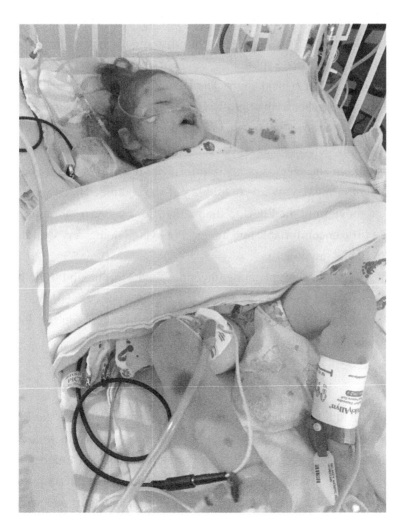

September 29, 2017

Our little miss Kendyl was doing well. She looked so good, especially considering that she just had a major surgery. It was fun to see her more awake. She kept asking for "wah wah" (water) and for "Alyx," which was touching. Her ultrasound showed good blood flow and her labs had already improved since before the surgery. Her IV (arterial line) and catheter were removed, and she received both blood and platelets that helped improve her skin color.

Through the afternoon and evening she was irritated and restless, and it was hard to see her like that. The oxygen in her nose was bugging her so she pulled it out constantly. She also did not like all the tubes (I don't blame her) and kept pulling on them. Already bored, she wanted to get back to her typical "hurricane Kendyl" ways. It was challenging and scary to see her trying to roll over, but it was great that she was well and wanted to move. I was able to hold her for a few minutes while they changed the sheets on her bed. I was nervous that I would hurt her incision, but she seemed pretty comfortable. It was wonderful and the highlight of my day. We were told that if she continued to do well, she would move from the PICU to the regular floor the next morning. She was a little uncomfortable and hungry but overall doing very well. I felt relieved and grateful.

It took some extra planning, meetings, and coordination to do both the bypass and the G-tube placement in the same surgery but was absolutely worth it. It is always nice to combine procedures, doctor appointments or trips to the hospital, when possible.

September 30, 2017

Kendyl had a few minor setbacks and was not able to leave the PICU as expected. However, she was doing well and continued to amaze me with how tough she was. Kids are amazing and much tougher than adults. She had been pretty irritable the previous day but did settle down for the night. She was also needing less pain medications and seemed to be more comfortable. Movies were a great distraction, especially *Frozen*. Anna, Elsa and Olaf were definitely helping us get through the hospital stay. She was now able to drink more water by mouth and she got started on Pedialyte through her G-tube. The doctors wanted to start her very slow (5 ml/hour), but she had been tolerating it well. Being able to have a little bit by mouth as well as through her tube helped calm her down. I knew she was hungry and that she was not used to this since she had been fed almost constantly through her NG tube until now.

It was amazing to watch the level of care Kendyl received from the team but especially from her surgeon. We were impressed to see him checking in frequently and using the surgery to teach others. While he had years of experience with this procedure, it was the first time it was done at this hospital. What an amazing timing it was to have him join the liver team just a few months before her surgery. Without his move, the surgery would have probably happened in Chicago. It was hard enough here, and I could not imagine what it would have been like to travel from Utah to Chicago for this procedure. This surgeon came at the perfect time, and I am sure his presence has blessed many other lives since.

October 2, 2017

Every day, Kendyl seemed to return more to her normal herself. There were some things that I had hoped she would forget that were coming back, such as saying, "mean mommy." I had been able to hold her more and more each day and each time it made me smile to watch her heart rate go down as I held her. Seeing her completely relax in my arms would melt my heart. She liked having me close and would cry when I left the room. It was sad to see her nervous and afraid of the nurses who were trying to take care of her, especially when I knew her fear was rooted in so much experience.

Kendyl cried all the way as we moved her from the PICU to the regular floor. She didn't understand that it was a good thing. The IV in her foot and the IJ (central line in her neck) were removed, and she would no longer require the oxygen support. A new peripheral IV was installed in her hand, in case they needed it. Her two bowel movements since her surgery were also a good sign. She was tolerating her formula well (now up to 15 ml/hour) and was also drinking a little more by mouth. The team had changed most of her meds from IV to mouth (which meant by tube in her case). We were grateful the tube was working well, and she was tolerating feeds.

Every time we were in the hospital, I felt bad for myself for a moment, but it did not take long to realize that others had it much worse. We were blessed to still have our child with us. I am sure that many would have traded places with us in a heartbeat if they could.

October 5, 2017

It was a day full of ups and downs. Kendyl's JP drain was removed, and she was meeting her feeding goals. She had been tolerating feeds well until she threw up her medications shortly before going to bed. I did not think much of it and assumed she would be fine the next day. However, she threw up again in the morning and had a fever. This was a disappointment because we were planning on going home that day. The good news was the ultrasound results looked great and her surgeon said the blood flow through the new vessel was beautiful. The bad news was we were still in the hospital.

Zach and I were both exhausted. One day in the hospital felt like the equivalent of three days at home. It was a hard and draining place to be. I always picked up some extra pounds each time, which was tough on my body. Trying to keep a positive attitude was challenging mentally. Controlling my temper, when I felt so frustrated, was hard emotionally. Watching your child go through so much, day after day, while having no idea how long it will last is unbearable.

Kendyl had two lab draws, two shots, one ultrasound, two X-rays and several checks of her vitals, and that was all in one day! It was hard to watch her not able to do things she could do just one week earlier, such as sitting, standing, and walking by herself. However, she was getting stronger every day. I was thrilled when I could hold her on my hip without her crying. I knew that once we returned home, she would have more determination to get where she was before. But until then, I needed to have patience and keep being there for her. Even with all the ups and downs, I was grateful and relieved that the surgery was over, and she was doing well overall.

I really had been terrified for this surgery and feared for the worst. It was a lot harder to hand our child over to the surgeons now that she was older, yet still young enough to not understand what was happening. I was grateful it was behind us. Her doctor now hoped the liver would be good for at least 20 years.

October 8, 2017

Primary Children's Hospital is amazing. I attended the small church service today and it was just as wonderful as I remembered. It was awesome that you could go in your sweats and that it was only 30–45 minutes. There was an amazing spirit that you could strongly feel, and it was humbling to hear testimonies from several people who had been through so much. They were full of strength, faith, and hope. There were not too many dry eyes because the spirit was so overwhelmingly strong.

It was also wonderful to have Carol F. McConkie, a church leader from the General Young Women's Board attend. She was the sweetest and the cutest and I marveled at her goodness. You could feel all the light and love she brought to the meeting. I believed there was a reason this hospital felt different than others and it was because of the powerful sprit present. They had so many wonderful leaders willing to help, pray, give blessings, or do anything they could to help lift those who had heavy burdens. I know without a doubt that God knew and loved every single child here, better than the nurses, the doctors, and even their parents. He was also aware of their families and current struggles. I am grateful for this knowledge and feeling that we are never alone.

If you ever get a chance to attend this amazing meeting, go! No matter what your faith is, I promise you will be touched.

October 9, 2017

I think it is safe to say we watched *Frozen* 100 times this week. Today Kendyl said, "Elsa on," meaning she wanted me to play the movie again. How could I say no to that? She was having a blood transfusion and it was quite difficult to keep her entertained and somewhat still for the process. This went on for a few long hours, but she breezed through it and remained happy. It was so great to see her get back to being herself. I am always amazed at how tough this special girl is. She had a great day in terms of how she was acting and playing, despite being poked so many times that I lost count. One of them happened when she only had 30 minutes of the transfusion left and we realized her IV had moved out of place, so she had to get a new one. Seriously?!

Even though she was going through so much, she was one happy girl. Hearing her laughing more and more was the sweetest sound. Seeing both my girls and my cute hubby made it a great day. Alyx kept saying she wanted her family to be together and I could not agree more. We all hoped to get "home" very soon. We didn't want to let Kendyl know this. It seemed that if she knew that she might be going home, she might have a fever, throw up, or something else to keep us there.

Kids are so strong. Never underestimate their resiliency.

October 10, 2017

We had a little bit of music therapy before being discharged and returning home. It was another 12 days in the hospital, but we were forever grateful for the positive impact the surgery had on our girl's little body. It was hard to see something permanent in her tummy, but it was also comforting to know we would not have traumatic moments

136

with the tube in her nose anymore. I was thankful that I wouldn't have to ever put that tube back in. That had been sad and stressful experiences for all of us!

Kendyl's numbers looked awesome; in fact, better than they had in several months. It is amazing to witness what surgery can do. She was now walking everywhere, tolerating feeds like a champ, even eating some chips here and there. Several days went by without needing any pain medications. Neither the G-tube nor the big incision were going to slow her down. Once again, we were so relieved and grateful for another huge blessing.

October 11, 2017

It felt like we had only been home for a few hours, and we already had to go in for early morning labs again. Luckily, we were able to go to McKay Dee Hospital, which was much closer. The girls both got little toy prizes for being good and they were happy about it. That morning, when I woke up Kendyl, she saw Alyx and immediately smiled, giggled, and said, "happy." It was so precious. There would be an adjustment period since our little warrior was on 24-hour feeds. She still wanted to walk, even though she was still a little weak and tipsy. It would be a busy week for me, chasing her around a messy house while carrying her formula bag, but it was so worth it! We all enjoyed being home altogether and sleeping in our own beds.

> Focus on what is truly important. (The dishes, the scattered toys, and the messy house can all wait.)

October 13, 2017

I felt overwhelmed by the long list of thank-you cards that I wanted to write, which is a great problem to have. My heart was full, and I was so thankful for all the things people had done for us. I was amazed by those willing to step up and be in service in times of need. People helped us with meals, with Alyx, with thoughtful gifts, messages, and many prayers. Some of those I know very well and others I barely knew. I really had been touched by so many people reaching out and letting us know they were thinking and praying for us. We definitely felt all the prayers received during this time. I wanted to write as many cards as possible, but I knew that I would not be able to thank everyone. I wished I could thank every person who said a prayer in our behalf. Same thing with all the families and companies who provided dinner at the Ronald McDonald Room at the hospital. Every single message, comment, and phone call to check in and see how we were doing meant a lot. Thank you. I promise that these acts of service, whether big or small, were appreciated.

October 19, 2017

It had only been three weeks since Kendyl's major surgery, but her incision was already looking awesome. The scar on her belly had been opened three separate times. And yet, it was crazy to see how far she had come; what a tough girl. Today we had an appointment at the hematology clinic to look at blood issues she had had in the past. We were told that she was doing great and that she would not need to be seen there again unless problems came back in the future.

At the doctor's office, I was once again humbled by others in the waiting room who were affected by various ailments or illnesses. Kendyl looked like the healthiest one in the room. Although I wish she could have been born with a perfect liver, I felt so thankful she didn't have something worse. She was doing well and looked so good that if you didn't notice the tube in her belly, you would have had no idea what she had been through.

I really cannot imagine what life would have been like without Kendyl's disease. I am sure that if I had two healthy girls, I would still be complaining about how hard motherhood is. God knew I had a lot to learn and that I would not have learned it another way. While I could not change the fact that she was born with a rare liver disease, I could decide to see the blessings, the tender mercies, the lessons, and be grateful that she was now kicking this disease to the curb.

October 21, 2017

My heart was filled with joy tonight as we took both girls to our church's trunk or treat. Alyx was the most beautiful Cinderella and her younger sister followed as the cutest Minnie Mouse. It was so great to watch Kendyl excited about this new experience. She was thrilled to be walking around, being outside and following Alyx wherever she went. She constantly smiled, giggled, and said thank you to each car. Many people were surprised to see her out and about and looking so good. When they asked how she was doing, I would respond that she was doing awesome and Kendyl would imitate me and say "awesome" in her cutest little voice. I was even thrilled to see her open a lollipop and chew on a wrapped candy bar on the way home. While we were driving home, Alyx kept saying how much fun it was to be there as a family. That night felt like a normal night for a little family with two healthy girls.

Treasure the simple but memorable moments.

October 26, 2017

Kendyl had her first follow-up visit with the liver team since her big surgery. A typical appointment meant leaving early, before she was given her medications, get lab work done, take her medications, and then see the liver team to discuss the lab results. They would usually go through the lab results with me, and I always recorded them in a little notebook that I could refer to. For the first time ever, they only said, "Everything looks great." The only number they discussed, which was not normal, was her GGT but they were not concerned about it. I immediately laughed and said, "Wow, going over her labs has never been this brief." The term I frequently heard from them was "stably elevated." Today was a different story as everything looked better.

They even showed us a graph and it was amazing to see how her body had responded since the procedure. I felt like bursting into tears of gratitude for her amazing surgeon. I appreciated that he was not only very talented and experienced with such a specific procedure, but he was also very personable. We even had his cell phone number as he had provided it when we first met. I took a picture of him and Kendyl that day and he asked me to send it to him. When I asked what had brought him here, he shared a little bit of his story. I was amazed by some details and happy to hear that moving his family here was good for them too. It truly was meant to be.

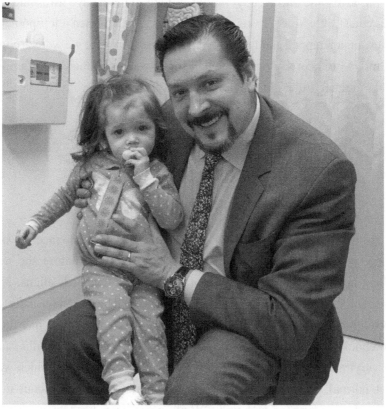

Kendyl with Dr. R.

October 29, 2017

We had two sleeping beauties on our bench during church service today. Even though it was hard trying to get all of us ready on Sunday mornings, it was so great to be there as a family. Since it was flu season, we did not take Kendyl to nursery but looked forward to her going back in the spring. Even if your kids are sleeping through church, not listening, being crazy, or anything else, it is always worth it to bring them.

One of my favorite quotes is "God loves effort," by President Russell M. Nelson.

October 31, 2017

I had really been looking forward to this day but unfortunately, it was not the Happy Halloween that I wanted it to be. We had such a fun day planned with lots of time together as a family. It started as a normal day but at 6 a.m. when I was about five minutes into my workout, Alyx came running downstairs and said, "Mommy you can't exercise. Kendyl is throwing up." I ran upstairs and sure enough she was right. After changing a few diapers, it was clear that she had some type of stomach bug. Because of this, I got Alyx to preschool a few mins late, again. I always felt bad when she was late because she did not want to miss anything. I came back home for a bit and then went to the lab and pharmacy before I rushed back to get Alyx. As I arrived at her school, I saw all the kids and their parents coming out. I somehow completely missed that I was supposed to be there for a performance. I felt so bad! Alyx was pretty good about it but on the way home she did say, "I kept calling for you mom." I was grateful that she was understanding, but it hurt to hear this.

After a few phone conversations with Kendyl's doctors, they wanted me to pick up a special probiotic for her that I could only get at the hospital. Since I was going to be down there, they wanted Kendyl examined by the wound clinic for granulation tissue around her G-tube.

Spending so much time in the car traveling and ending it at the hospital wasn't the fun holiday I thought it would be. There are times when we might feel like we are failing in every aspect of our lives. That's when we need to remind ourselves that tomorrow is a new day.

November 7, 2017

The first few weeks with the G-tube were a little hard. For the first six weeks, it really stuck out and seemed to get in the way. We had to watch her closely so that she did not pull it out. If she ever pulled it out in the first six weeks, we would need to get her to the ER quickly to have it put back in. We were constantly cleaning around the tube site, using tape to keep it in place, and watching her closely. We were lucky to get through the critical part without a trip to the emergency room. It was quite a process, but my girl now had a G-tube button. Her tube was in and now more permanent.

We had decided to celebrate a new milestone with our little miss having a real bath the next day. I felt so grateful for being persistent in getting her the tube as it was the best decision. Since most patients thrive after a transplant, her liver doctor was not too familiar with G-tubes. Kendyl was also one of the first liver transplant patients to have one. At the time it felt like the G-tube was a step backwards. However, this step was the right decision that we needed to make for our girl to move forward.

In life we take steps forward and backward.
At times, the steps backwards are necessary
for us to be able to move forward.

Fall of 2017

I was terrified the first time Kendyl pulled out her G-tube. I was upstairs cleaning the bathroom when Alyx came to tell me something was wrong. Sure enough, she was right, and I initially panicked. I didn't want to bother Zach at work, but I felt like I needed some help.

Without really thinking about it (I hate to ask for help), I quickly called my nurse friend who lives down the street. After I asked if she was home and available to help me, she said she would be right over. She came moments later and was happy to help. While she was not super familiar with G-tubes, she reassuringly told me that we would figure it out together. I found something on my phone to keep Kendyl distracted as I gathered the supplies that I needed to put the tube back in. This included a syringe, distilled water, gauze, and a new button (it sits on top of the stomach where the tube is hooked in for feedings). As my friend sat next to me, my mind was suddenly very clear. I was calm and able to place the tube back in. I was so relieved to see how easy it was. I am still grateful that she was home that day and able to come over right away. She did not feel like she did much to help, but she did.

Sometimes we think we need to do something big to help others. While big things might be great, sometimes small things mean just as much, if not more. That day I needed help to put the tube back in as I didn't feel qualified to do it, but because of her calming manner, I was able to do it by myself. She brought me some peace and allowed me to calm down so I could think clearly and fix the problem. I am not even sure my friend remembers this day but if she does, she would probably say it was not a big deal, but it was to me. Little things really do make a big difference.

November 12, 2017

It was my beautiful sister's wedding day. A very special day. After a heartbreaking divorce right after having her first baby, she was getting married again and it was so exciting. Weddings are always special, but I remember how cute and healthy Kendyl looked, and it made the day mean so much more. It now felt like we had closed the chapter on hospital visits and surgeries. Watching my sister marry the man who had helped heal her heart filled me with joy. I was also grateful to see both of our girls running around and enjoying this memorable day.

December 1, 2017

This night turned out differently than we had planned. We had plans to meet Zach after work and take the girls to see the Christmas lights in Ogden. Kendyl wasn't feeling well so instead I spent the whole afternoon holding her and giving her lots of snuggles. This made up for fun plans that did not happen. We did not have "plans" very often so canceling them made it hard and more frustrating. When Zach came home, I had a meltdown. I was sad, angry, overwhelmed, and exhausted. As I expressed my feelings with him, I let the tears flow. I felt really bad for Alyx because she had been so excited to see the Christmas lights, and she was going to miss out on another activity because of her sister. That's when Alyx came right over to me and said, "mommy, it is OK. We can go another time. I am OK." A few moments later she started praying that Kendyl would feel better. It melted my heart. Sometimes, as a parent, I feel like I have lots to teach my kids, but they also keep teaching me so much. Those little moments are so precious and priceless. As we got the girls to bed, I quoted a well-known line in our family, picked up from my grandma Jones, "I thought tonight would be more fun." Although it was different than expected, it was a moment that meant a lot. It warmed my heart more than seeing some Christmas lights.

December 11, 2017

Kendyl was still feeling sick. She had been getting better, but it was obvious she didn't feel well. After a short liver clinic visit, the doctors wanted her to be admitted. Her lab results showed that she had three viruses and still had C. diff (she had had it off and on for months). The liver numbers were still off but were better than they had been a few weeks prior. Because of the viruses, she had also developed pneumonia and was struggling to breathe so she needed some oxygen. Luckily, it was a short hospital stay, and she came home two days later. We were so grateful that she would be home before Christmas.

December 19, 2017

Alyx and I delivered books with notes on them to Primary Children's Hospital for them to give to children on Christmas Day. She had helped me tie a little ribbon around each one with a note that read, "Merry Christmas from a little family who was in the hospital one year for Christmas. Thinking of you." It was fun to be able to talk with her about the year Kendyl was admitted during the holiday and have a teaching moment about why we did this. I was impressed to see how much more she understood compared with the previous year. It was precious to hear her tell Kendyl that the books were not for them but for kids in the hospital and how she hoped it would make them happy. It was not much (there were only 24 books in total) but it was such a fun memory. This has become a cherished tradition for our family as we understand how difficult it is to spend holidays in that environment. We want to give back and share the spirit of Christmas in some small way with those who have to spend it away from home.

Make fun traditions and do not let
teaching moments pass by.

December 2017

The 12 days of Christmas were magical for us that year. Someone sweet, thoughtful, and kind anonymously brought little pieces of a darling Fisher-Price nativity set each day. Our family looked forward to the knock every night and tried a few times to peek, but we have never been able to figure out who it was. It brought such a sweet feeling into our home, and we will always remember it. I would give almost anything to know who the sweet individual or family was so I could say, "THANK YOU." I wish I could express to them how much this has meant to us. It is a memory we will hold dear for years to come.

The girls love the nativity set and continue to enjoy it each year when we get our Christmas decorations out. I am grateful for so many Christlike people in my life both near and far. There is such a special spirit at Christmas time.

December 21, 2017

I felt like I had been witnessing a miracle this week. Not only did Kendyl's labs look absolutely perfect (the best they had looked in a long time or possibly ever). She had also been eating so much better by mouth! She was very interested in what everyone was eating (especially Alyx) and wanted to try just about anything. Throughout the week she had eaten a little bit of pretzels, carrots, chips, a lollipop, rice, apples, bread, sweet potatoes, goldfish crackers, bananas, Cheerios, and M&M's. This was an amazing milestone for her.

I continued to pray, hope and keep my fingers crossed this would continue. It definitely seemed that when she felt good, she ate more, and this was probably the best she had ever felt in her entire life. She had a healthy liver, with normal portal vein flow and she was now over her viruses and pneumonia. I was hoping that we could keep her healthy so she could continue moving in the right direction. This was the best Christmas present!

December 25, 2017

It was a special Christmas day. I do not remember what gifts were given or received but I remember the joy of the day. After being in the hospital for Christmas in 2015 and then living with my parents for Christmas in 2016, it was exciting to have our own home and celebrate with our little family.

Chapter 4
LiveReal
2018

January 23, 2018

K endyl had another clinic appointment with her amazing liver doctor. It was a very uneventful visit, which is just the way we like them. She was still tiny (23.5 lb) and was in the 6th percentile for height and 5th percentile for weight, but she was doing well. We were also able to meet a social media friend in person who had had a transplant four years earlier. It was fun to see older kids doing well and living mostly normal lives. This gave us so much hope and peace for Kendyl's future. I also enjoyed how these appointments changed over time. Prior to her transplant, I would sit on the edge of my seat and cling to every word they would say. I always had a bag packed just in case she was admitted, and I would also wonder and worry about how much time she had left. These all seemed to be things of the past as she had recently begun to show us that she was in the "terrible twos," but I was grateful for this experience.

January 26, 2018

Before I had kids, I could imagine being a perfect mom to my four kids. They were healthy and happy, my house was clean, and I was always put together both inside and out. I was a happy mom who never felt overwhelmed, and I definitely never yelled. Maybe you were a perfect parent before you had kids too. However, now that I have kids, this perfect picture is not reality.

Kendyl was tired and I put her down for a nap. Because she drank so much during the day, we had up to ten blankets and towels in her bed at all times to protect the mattress. After quite some time had gone by, I could still hear her clearly not sleeping and decided to check on her. I found her in her crib jumping and laughing, with all the blankets on the outside of the crib, her pants and diaper off. She had peed on the bed (thank goodness she could not get the mattress cover off or it would have been ruined). I also found her diaper on the floor completely dry.

After I cleaned her up and the bed, put new blankets, and laid her down, I yelled for her to go sleep. She eventually did but it was after some of the saddest cries I've ever heard. I sat on my bed for a moment, so mad at myself for getting angry with her. How could I do that? I felt guilty for behaving the way I did and feared that she might hate me forever. I especially felt bad that we had almost lost her before the transplant and here I was treating her this way. I did not respond the way I should have, but I was also tired and frustrated. Motherhood is hard and exhausting. I once heard something that describes it perfectly, "The days are long, but the years are short."

Even if your kids have been through traumatic experiences, and even if you have almost lost them, you are still human. It's normal to react in ways you might not be proud of.

February 26, 2018

Kendyl was not feeling her best, which always made me feel exhausted and helpless as a momma. The morning started early with labs and two pokes that were so traumatic that they left blood on my pants, along with many tears. When we got home Kendyl cried, and I was not able to console her. She finally calmed down a little after some Tylenol but still wanted me to hold her constantly. She would only sleep on me and if I tried to lay her down, she woke up and cried.

I called her liver doctor to check on her lab results and they were a little off. I knew they weren't going to be great based on how she was feeling. When they asked how she was doing, I told them she was definitely not herself. I also told them that she had a bad fall on the tile the night before. She had tripped on a bar stool and landed right on the back of her head. They were a bit more concerned about her not feeling well because she was taking aspirin as a blood thinner, so they wanted her to be checked out. We headed to the ER, wondering how long we would be there this time. Luckily, it wasn't too long, and she was OK. She had a virus with a fever, so they had to cancel the CT scan scheduled for the next day, but at least we knew everything was well.

March 7, 2018

It had been a very long 24 hours. Kendyl had been sick for several weeks with a cold she could not seem to kick and had spiked a fever of 102 during the night. I called the doctor who was on call hoping I could take her into her pediatrician the next day but was told to bring her to the ER.

As we arrived, she didn't look good. She was breathing fast and heavy, had a fever, and was really pale. I was quite certain she had pneumonia since she had it only a few months prior. She was immediately taken back to a room for labs, tests, and a chest X-ray. The tests showed she had three viruses: rhino virus (common cold), adenovirus, and RSV and she also had a little bit of pneumonia.

We were admitted and finally got settled in a room around 3 a.m. I had been up since 5 a.m. the previous morning so I was exhausted. After a few hours of rest, we had a day full of playing, giggles, and laughing. I kept thinking that I should remind her that she was sick. It made me laugh that one of her favorite things to say at the time was "I tricked you" which was very fitting. She was often a mystery, even to her doctors.

Although it was hard to be in the hospital each time, I was always humbled. I was reminded of a much bigger picture. It was hard to care for her most of the time, but at least we were home and not living in the hospital for long periods. Our inpatient visits were becoming less frequent, shorter, and not as serious as they once were. I was grateful for this.

So many memories and emotions came up as we got in the same room we were in when we first came two years prior. It was quite a whirlwind being discharged from the Spokane Hospital and flying to Salt Lake, but I still remember many of the emotions and fears. I felt grateful to be where we were today, knowing that Kendyl would be going home the next day, and that once again it was a short stay.

We can be triggered by little things. It is OK
to let them bring up emotions but don't spend
too much time dwelling there.

March 30, 2018

I felt the Lord's hand in our lives over the past week. We received the news that Alyx had been accepted to a charter school where we had hoped she would begin kindergarten in the fall. I felt a sense of relief about her attending this school rather than the public one she would have otherwise. I was not ready to let her go to full-day kindergarten, and I knew she would miss a lot of school with Kendyl still having so many early lab days. I was feeling so grateful that Alyx could now go to a great school in the afternoons, which was best for all of us. This would push us another year past the transplant, which we hoped would mean fewer early morning lab trips by the time she was in first grade and going all day.

We received another huge hospital bill but thankfully a reimbursement came from a foundation that helped with medical expenses. We were so fortunate to have insurance and foundations helping us with her medical bills. I hoped that someday we could give back to help others in similar circumstances.

Spring of 2018

There had been times when I wondered why we had gone to school so far away from home and why we moved 700 miles away from all family. However, we met amazing people while we were in Spokane that we would never have had the chance to meet if we hadn't moved there.

I met one of my beautiful friends, whom I will never forget, at a church meeting, right after moving to Spokane. It was our first Sunday there all by ourselves (the week before my parents were there helping us move in). She introduced herself and it meant so much to know that the "pretty girl" (I couldn't remember her name) might want to be my friend. I was insecure and struggling at the time, so the move was really hard. This simple gesture meant the world to me and from then on, she continued to be my friend. My favorite moments were our runs/walks in the morning and our talks during that time. I cannot describe how much I needed it as there were so many reasons. She was an amazing friend and always had such a positive attitude that I admired.

It has been a few years since we moved back to Utah, and we still keep in touch with many of the wonderful people we met in Spokane. I was recently able to see some of those friends while they were in Utah visiting family. I was grateful that they made time to visit us during their family vacation. The people we met in Spokane will always have a special place in my heart. We were blessed to have that chapter in our lives.

Don't miss out on opportunities to meet amazing people. Some will leave lasting impacts.

April 9, 2018

I received a call from Make-A-Wish about a once-in-a-lifetime opportunity for our family. This brought me to tears and I had thoughts, such as "we don't deserve that" and "another family probably deserves it more." It was interesting to notice my thoughts changing so rapidly. Life can be hard for so long and then when it changes, we quickly forget how bad it really was. This was now the case for me.

Everything started when I was pregnant with Kendyl and got very sick. Then she was born and diagnosed with a life-threatening disease. We went through a sudden move, a transplant, and a period of uncertainty while trying to find a job. This was followed by hospital stays, many tests, tears, fears, procedures and many struggles.

Zach now had a job that he loved, we had a home, Kendyl was doing better, Alyx was settled and adjusted to life, and I had a new purpose and passion for taking care of myself. We often talked about how well things were going for us. If only we could have seen our future when life was so difficult, it would have been easier to live through the trying times. We would have loved to know that life would not just be OK, that it would be wonderful. I probably would not have stressed so much about the future when we were in the hospital.

Because life was now good, I felt guilty for the amazing opportunity that was being offered to our family. I tried to embrace it by remembering that life had been hard for a long time (several years). It was a blessing that the hard memories were already fading. I have learned that we don't grow much when life's path is easy.

Whether you are in a good chapter or a not-so-great chapter of life, keep going.

April 16, 2018

It was a tiring day, which was usual when Kendyl had an appointment with her liver team, but it felt different as we hadn't been there in a couple of months. Her labs were a little off, so the doctors wanted a biopsy to check her liver, which we scheduled a few weeks out. The team kept commenting on how great she looked. At every appointment her doctor reminded us how sick she had been before the transplant. I was so grateful, happy, and pleased with how she was doing. She still had the G-tube and life was not completely "normal" but we had come a long way.

I was so appreciative for Kendyl's liver team. Although I wished our girl had not been born with an awful disease, I can't imagine not knowing all of them. With any journey, whether health related or not, having a caring team to cheer you on makes a big difference. I told the team today, "You all said it would get easier the longer out from the transplant, but I didn't believe you. However, I am starting to, now." Not only was the team wonderful for Kendyl, but the hospital was great with Alyx as well. At each appointment, Alyx would go to the "fun place," as she called it, where they would watch her. She would play with toys and Playdough, paint, do crafts, watch movies and more. Alyx would look forward to these days, which helped so much. The only time Kendyl cried that day was while we were picking up Alyx. She started playing with a big green dinosaur and had to let go of it as we were leaving. I felt blessed to be surrounded with so many good people on the journey, especially those who helped make it fun for Alyx.

Everyone has a different journey. Find people who will support you no matter what journey you are on.

April 18, 2018

Kendyl finally had a CT scan. We had been trying to get it done for months and it was rescheduled three times because she was sick. It was a long day, but I was glad they were able to finally do it. I was not really worried about these results. As they were prepping Kendyl for sedation, the nurse had read her chart and said, "She is a complex kiddo." Although it was hard to hear, I definitely agreed. Her journey had not been easy, but she continued to fight through each obstacle.

April 23, 2018

This was the National Pediatric Transplant Week. Reflecting on it, so many thoughts came up which I recorded in my journal.

> *"As we get further out from transplant (it will be two years in July), I lose a little bit more hope of hearing from the donor family... As a mom I can't help but wonder the gender of the child, the age of the child, and the location of where the child was from. In my head I have an idea for all of these, but I am probably wrong. The only thing we know for sure is that it was about an hour flight away. I would give anything to hear from them and meet them if they were open to it...*
>
> *I remember as we started the transplant evaluation process, the surgeon said something like, 'the right organ seems to find the right recipient.' At the time I thought 'Oh that's cool' but as I pondered it more, I couldn't shake the thought because now I believe that with all my heart to be true because of my faith. I believe our Heavenly Father knew which organ was best for Kendyl and which one would end up being the one for her. Before the actual surgery, she was an alternate twice and we had one false alarm. At the time we were devastated but I believe those didn't work out for a reason."*

April 29, 2018

It was an eventful Sunday. Zach and I were able to go to church together with Alyx. I was glad that we could be there together while a family member was watching Kendyl at home. We were grateful we could see a new bishop (church leader of our congregation) be called. We loved both the previous and the new one as well.

For the second hour of church, I was scheduled to teach the women. We were wrapping up the song before the lesson when the newly called Bishop came in and told me that Zach was trying to get a hold of me. I usually didn't check my phone in church, so I had no idea. He told me that Kendyl had pulled out her G-tube out and Zach needed help. I rushed home and we were able to get it back in before I quickly went back to the church to teach the lesson. Although I was a little frazzled, I was able to get through it. Thankfully, it didn't take long, and the women were understanding. We were already putting our new bishop to work.

May 1, 2018

We had such a wonderful night as a family. We went to the Make-A-Wish office in Murray, Utah, where we discussed possibilities for Kendyl's wish. There were so many options. Some of the more interesting ones were a shopping spree, a nice playground (that sounded amazing, but we were currently renting) and a trip. Kendyl was hard to keep entertained as she walked around everywhere. We put in a few options for family trips, with our first choice being Disney World in Orlando, Florida. The timing for this meeting was perfect as we anticipated going in for a biopsy the next day to see why her numbers continued to climb. I felt so much gratitude that night for my little family, for this opportunity, and wondered how I was so blessed.

May 2, 2018

There was not much sleep that night as I had to switch Kendyl's tube feeds in the middle of night from formula to water so she could be fasting. I felt so bad waking her up when she was sleeping so peacefully but we had to leave the house at 5:30 a.m. for an early arrival time. The liver biopsy went well and there were no signs of bleeding. She handled the anesthesia well and bounced back quickly after she woke up. She remained under observation for several hours, so we spent the afternoon snuggling (I loved that she had a big bed), watching movies, and playing with play dough. It was a long day as we got home around 5 p.m., yet grateful that we were not admitted. We were told that we may have to go back the next day depending on the results of the biopsy.

I was hoping, praying, and keeping my fingers crossed it was not her body rejecting the liver.

May 4, 2018

We finally heard back and the results from the biopsy showed there was no rejection! We were thrilled and relieved. However, the clinic was a little concerned that the blood flow through the vessel that was put in last fall (Rex Bypass Surgery) might be worse than they thought. It was hard to hear that news and we were amazed that our little baby just continued to fight through hurdles. She was getting sassier by the day and continued to teach and inspire me.

The future was a still unknown for our girl, but we kept our fingers crossed that all would be well. With all the prayers on Kendyl's behalf, it felt like we could make it through whatever might come our way. We continued to hold to our faith.

May 5, 2018

The girls and I had a fun day at the Discovery Gateway Museum for kids. It was Alyx's last preschool field trip, and I was grateful that I could go and help. Her favorite activities were being a construction worker and telling all the other kids what to do. It felt great to get out and it was fun to watch the girls play and explore.

As I watched them play, I could not help but see two cute girls, two sisters, playing. I realized for the first time that no one around would know what these girls had been through. Kendyl seemed like a normal tiny two and a half-year old. I had given her a feed on the way down and left the bag in the car while we played. No one knew she was a transplant kiddo and had a tube in her belly. It was a refreshing sight that warmed my heart, and it gave me a glimpse of how things would hopefully be in the future. I had wished for life to be like this so long and thought it might never happen. Although it was complete chaos, chasing them both by myself and losing them a few times, it was a great day and we all made it home safely. I had debated taking Kendyl along because of the fear that her suppressed immune system might be facing too many germs, but it was worth it. I felt like a lucky (and tired) momma. Holding on to the hope of how things might be in the future is always worthwhile.

May 21, 2018

Today's clinic appointment felt a little unsettling as we discussed Kendyl's blood flow issue with the clotted portal vein. I asked so many questions that day. Did they think the small balloon procedure they mentioned would work? Would she need another big surgery? Was it OK to wait a bit to do it with me going out of town (which I told them I could cancel) or should we do it now? A lot of options were discussed without many "for sure" answers. We decided that she was okay to wait, and we scheduled the small balloon procedure for early July.

When I went to pick up Alyx from the "fun place," they asked if we would be interested in going to the zoo and told me that they had saved some tickets for us. The main care leader knew us well because we were there so much. It was such a blessing because at that moment I was trying to keep it together and not cry. Kendyl's visit had been heavy and sad. This woman didn't know any of this, but I truly felt it was a way of letting me know that God was there and aware of me and my family that day.

June 1, 2018

We had a wonderful night as a family at the Hogle Zoo. It was a special event for families who had children with health challenges. It was nice to fit right in as many of us had the same feeding tube pump and bag. Yet, I was once again reminded of how lucky we were and that our situation could be much worse. We were able to meet Cinderella, Belle, and Rapunzel. The girls loved it! It was a night we all needed.

Getting out with others in a similar
situation brings comfort.

June 2, 2018

My sister and I went on a shopping spree to get me some summer clothes. I had very few due to many reasons: Law school, being pregnant, having most of my clothes packed away, Kendyl's transplant, money being tight, and other things that came along the way. Over the last few summers, I had just lived in t-shirts and sweats. My mom had even mentioned that she remembered a year when I wore sweats all summer.

I felt so grateful to be where we were; life was a little more settled, money was not as tight, and Kendyl was so much more stable. I finally felt like I could get away for a few hours and get new things to wear that summer.

June 2018

We met with an ENT (Ear, Nose and Throat) doctor who had been referred to us by the feeding therapist. He suspected that Kendyl had been aspirating, so he wanted to do a swallow study within the next few weeks. This issue was something we would have never picked up on without our amazing therapist. A few days later, an ultrasound was done to look at the blood flow of the donor vessel that had been placed in September. We had been watching it closely for a few weeks. The procedure went well and was actually one of the easiest ones. The tech was fast and thorough and Kendyl was holding still. However, the results came back as we expected. The flow was not great, so she was going to have a procedure to correct it in a few weeks.

The date had been changed several times and we still didn't have a "for sure" date in place. Working things out with schedules of multiple doctors was challenging.

Kendyl's condition continued to raise stress, worry, and exhaustion. For me it seemed to bring acne breakouts and a short temper. Her condition often made me want to just "shut down," however, I couldn't. I wanted to be available for my family.

June 15, 2018

We hit a new milestone when Kendyl was able to eat something in the car. To most people this does not seem like a big deal, but it was huge for us. I had not felt comfortable letting her eat in the car previously because she choked so easily. She only had a few nibbles (which is typical) and she didn't choke at all. It was exciting!

June 20–23, 2018

From the moment when Kendyl was diagnosed, it felt as though my days had been completely focused on her and Alyx. I had given up on doing anything for me, like running or having close friends. I had convinced myself that our difficult situation was going to last forever. I loved being a mom! It was an honor to have that title and I was grateful for my girls, but it was hard.

Thankfully, I had found an outlet through health and fitness. I had heard about the Summit Event conference, which sounded fun and amazing. For a long time, I wondered if I would ever really be able to attend but I now felt this was my year to go. I registered, bought my plane tickets and was looking forward to attending this event with my sister. At some point, I thought that I might need to postpone this to another year because of Kendyl's blood flow issue but her team told me that her procedure could wait and that I should go. I was relieved and excited that I could still go to the event in Indianapolis. I remember a family member asking if I knew where that was, I laughed and said, "Uh … no … but I don't care… I'm going." That is a true story.

The theme of the event was "Believe in You." It was a beautiful and important theme that everyone should embrace. It made me wonder how the world would be different if we all believed in ourselves. There are so many people in the world, me included, who feel as though we are not good enough, not doing enough, or feel that we are not making a difference. God knows we can do incredible things when we believe in ourselves and in others.

During the event I heard a line that hit my heart very strongly. "This opportunity saves mommies." My eyes instantly teared up because I was one of those mommies. I had truly been saved by my new focus on my health, happiness, passion and purpose.

The most memorable experience of the event was finishing a 1.5-hour workout in the heat with amazing ladies and moms. I'm so happy that my sister was celebrating this experience with me. As I finished and we took pictures in the street, the tears flowed. I was grateful to realize that I was a mom, but also now a part of something amazing. I was helping mommies. I was now part of a community that was indescribable. Besides my faith and my family, I hadn't ever been a part of something so meaningful.

Attending that event was even more powerful than I thought it could possibly be. The emotions that were felt were truly transformational. Many giggles, tears, hugs, and memories were made. The journey attracted so many great people into my life and friendships that I didn't know I needed. It brought so much peace, hope, and happiness to a mom with a heavy heart. I loved having the opportunity to help others just like I had been helped. This trip ended up being the first of many as I began attending this event each year. It is now something that the whole family is used to. I look forward to going each year and the girls enjoy spending time with Dad like they did that year. The choices we make do not just affect us, they impact our families and those around us. If you are not motivated to do it for yourself, think of those around you. Knowing that my kids are watching me gives me the motivation to always keep going and be the best possible version of me.

It always seemed like a good idea to take care of myself, but after Kendyl's diagnosis, it became something I had to do to handle what was ahead of us. Being healthy looks and feels different for everyone. Some want six-pack abs, some want toned muscles, etc. I want those too but what is most important to me is how I FEEL. I want to feel strong, happy, and good, not only physically but mentally and emotionally as well. This isn't only important for mommas with sick babies, but for everyone in general. I honestly don't think we would have survived without me being forced to learn this lesson. I am blessed to be able to do something I LOVE while being home with my girls who bring so much joy to my life. I hope I can be the best version of myself every day for them.

The greatest gift you can give your family
and the world is a healthy you.

June 2018

I was doing the dishes one morning after returning from my trip and Alyx said to me out of the blue, "Mom, don't give up on your dreams. I believe in you." I was completely caught off guard, but it touched my heart and brought such a huge smile to my face. I have heard the statement that the demons we don't face we leave for our kids. The first time I heard that I gasped a little and then as I thought about it, I realized how true it was. Even though I hadn't intentionally told her of my goals and dreams, she had heard me talk about them with Zach and had picked up on them. I was grateful for her innocent and sweet reminder. I hope that she will remember her mom going after her dreams and that she will do the same.

Our kids are watching. If we don't chase our dreams
what does that teach them about their
own goals and aspirations?

July 2, 2018

Kendyl had a big day … early morning labs at one hospital, and then a liver clinic appointment at another one in the afternoon. She now weighed 12.3 kilos or 27 lb! The team just kept saying she looked so good and big. In fact, we were told to cut back a daily feed and she had outgrown the dose of one of her meds.

We were thrilled that she was growing well, but also tried to stay calm as we prepared for her balloon procedure in a few days. The small procedure, performed in radiology, would blow up the portal vein vessel to hopefully increase blood flow. Kendyl had previous procedures done in radiology and I felt good about the doctor who would be performing it. Her labs looked OK, which to us implied that the blood vessel was fine and that they just needed to improve the blood flow. We were confident that the procedure would be successful.

Kendyl was two weeks away from her liver-anniversary. Again, this was not how we had pictured her journey at this milestone, but we prepared and hoped it would be the last procedure she would need for a while.

July 4, 2018

It was not the typical July 4th U.S. holiday that we were used to. The day was busy cleaning and preparing for Kendyl's early procedure the next day. Although we didn't celebrate much, we reflected and were grateful for our freedom. That night we went to bed early and hoped that the fireworks would be kept to a minimum so we could all get some sleep. We were grateful the girls were little and didn't know what they were missing.

July 5, 2018

Zach and I arrived at the hospital early. Alyx stayed with my grandma for the night which made things easier in the morning. Even though it was a small procedure, it was still hard to place our little one in someone else's hands. We said goodbye to Kendyl after watching them put her to sleep and then went to the waiting room. We had mentally prepared for a long procedure, and we actually hoped for it because that would mean they had found the blood vessel and could attempt to insert the "balloon" to make it bigger. Luckily, we had some of our family with us, so we were able to talk and laugh as we waited.

It hadn't been very long, just as I had pulled out a book to read, when Dr. F. came out with Dr. R. I thought that they were coming to give me an update, which I thought was strange so early in the procedure. However, it wasn't an update. My heart sunk as Dr. F., the radiologist, said, "I am so sorry. I can't find it." I could not believe it. The tears started flowing and I could not turn them off.

I felt like my "mother's intuition" was usually spot on and I was really confident that the procedure would be a success. Unfortunately, I was wrong. As I continued to cry, Kendyl's surgeon put his hand on my back and said something like "It isn't what we wanted but it will be OK." He was as amazing outside the operating room as he was inside. We could tell he felt bad and had true empathy for what we were going through. The other doctor also kindly told us that he was sorry. I don't remember who was near the waiting room that day, except for family and the doctors, but I am sure that I made a scene. Shortly after, Kendyl was admitted under observation to make sure there was no internal bleeding. She had several small pokes on her chest from attempts to find the vessel.

It was the first time being admitted in a room with a twin-size bed instead of a crib, which allowed me to snuggle her. That was exactly what I needed at the moment. We were told that she would have to stay for one night. Our family stayed for most of the day and Kendyl became more awake and aware as the anesthesia wore off. My mind raced to know what our plan would be now. The doctors told me again not to worry and that everything would be OK.

I found it interesting that in the few short minutes when I had cracked open my book in the waiting room earlier, I had read about

God's timing and how it might be different from ours. That, to me, was not a coincidence. Of all the messages I could have read in that short amount of time, it was exactly what I needed to know that day.

July 6, 2018

The next morning the team did their morning rounds and started talking about ammonia. At the time I didn't even know what that was. I recall it had been mentioned a few times briefly before the Rex Bypass the year before, but it hadn't been a big concern, so I didn't look into it. I started asking questions and was told that ammonia is the amount of protein in your blood. At the time there was no reason to check it, but Kendyl's doctor just wanted to be sure. Her level was 100 and they wanted it less than 50. The doctors were surprised it was so high so they thought it must have been a fluke and not an accurate number. Checking ammonia is a sensitive test where the blood must go on ice immediately after being drawn. They assumed that maybe the high number had something to do with how the test had been done, so they wanted another one just to be sure. The second test came at 101! We were all shocked. It felt like another punch to the gut. How could this be?

I remember sitting outside Kendyl's room as the team showed me some options we could try to bring that number down. Some were really expensive, but we were willing to try whatever we could. The initial plan was to not do anything right now, except for changes in her diet to reduce protein intake, and keep watching her labs. The team felt confident that with nutrition and medication changes the level would improve.

It was a blessing that the doctor had decided to check Kendyl's ammonia level because she had shown no symptoms of a high level. Once again, I felt grateful for her whole team. Her surgeon, the radiology doctor, her liver doctor, and her liver team were all involved in the event of the day and concerned with the discouraging news.

We were discharged a few hours later. It was a weird feeling going home as the whole experience had gone completely different than I had imagined. It felt like we now had a whole new serious issue to deal with. We rushed home to see Alyx attending a little graduation from an online preschool program she had completed.

Sometimes life doesn't go as planned. No matter how much you want something, and regardless of how many prayers you and others have said.

July 14, 2018

Zach and I had such a fun night. He had surprised me a few months earlier with tickets to see Keith Urban who is my absolute favorite. It was so good to get out and enjoy some time with just the two of us. I thoroughly enjoyed the night, which included paying for an overpriced, but well worth, t-shirt and singing my little heart out in the heat. It was great!

At the end of this amazing concert, Keith thanked everyone for coming. He briefly mentioned the sacrifices some went through to be there, such as distance, money, getting sitters for kids, etc. He was sincere (I've seen him enough to know this is typical) and said that it would have been easier to do nothing than do those things to be there. The babysitter part really stuck out to me because it took some work getting everything ready for my parents and sister to watch the girls. We had a practice run and three pages of notes. In a lot of ways, it would have been easier to do "nothing" and stay home and not go. However, I was so glad we went and grateful to my family for their help.

Once we arrived home, my mom told us that Kendyl had pulled out her tube again. It was the one thing she was worried most about and just as she feared, it happened. She called the same friend who had helped me the first time and this amazing soul came to help put the tube back in without any problems. We were again grateful for my friend's help and for my mom being willing to watch the girls.

> It is often easier to do nothing. However, we miss out
> on a lot when we decide to follow the easiest path.
> The effort is usually worth it.

July 18, 2018

Kendyl had a swallow study, and I was really nervous about it. She was so picky with flavors and actually preferred things with no flavor. I wondered how I would convince her to drink the chalky liquid. Thankfully, it went better than I anticipated, as far as her cooperating. However, the results revealed that her swallowing issues were worse than we thought. She aspirated (meaning that liquids went to her lungs) with all fluids, regardless of the consistency (half nectar, nectar, and even honey, which is the thickest). It was hard to hear how bad her situation was and that we had another issue to be concerned about. We knew that this would mean additional doctor appointments and therapy.

As hard as it was to hear the results, I was more grateful than ever for her feeding tube. Based on the quantity of fluids required to flush her kidneys, there was no way she could have consumed her minimum goal of 43 oz by mouth, especially when she required so much thickener. That amount would not quench her thirst and it would also cause her to be constipated. As we went through this hurdle, we realized that it would be a while before she could get rid of her feeding tube. From this point on, we gave her about 8 oz of thickened water for her to drink during the day, and the rest of her fluid would go through the tube without the thickener.

It was interesting to notice what was happening. While she needed the tube when it was placed in September of 2017, she needed it even more now. I was once again reminded of why I felt the strong intuition to have her get the G-tube at that time.

Sometimes you might get a deeper understanding about a situation later and realize why you felt so strongly about it.

July 20, 2018

It was a rough week with lots of tears. Although we had just celebrated Kendyl's two-year liver anniversary, we were still a little crushed about the swallow study results and her ammonia level now reaching 137, which was more than double what they wanted it to be.

As the team discussed her best options, different surgeries were mentioned along with the possibility of another transplant. I was not prepared for them to bring this up. They made it clear that a second transplant would be the last resort and it wouldn't be happening any time soon, but the fact that it was mentioned made my stomach hurt. Everything felt so up and down, and this roller coaster was not as fun as the awesome rides I used to like. We would know more with time, but based on the latest information, the anxious feelings I was getting from everyone on the medical team, the fact that we were meeting with them so often (about every two weeks) and having more labs (up to twice a week), I felt defeated, sad and angry.

I had so many thoughts going through my mind, such as why did she have to go through so much? Why is she experiencing so many complications, both related and unrelated to the liver transplant? How am I ever going to be strong enough to keep being there for her? I felt too young to go through these challenges. Maybe my parents could handle something like this, but not me. I had never pictured such a scenario, two years post-transplant.

Even with my heavy heart, the constant pit in my stomach, and the feeling that I could burst into tears without notice, I still knew that things could be worse and that we were blessed. I had the sweetest husband who was there for me, who listened, let me cry, made me laugh, and reminded me that we were in this together and that we would make it through these upcoming hurdles.

Life is quite the ride. Do your best to enjoy it.

July 28, 2018

"A family that has haircuts together stays together." OK, maybe that is not an actual saying but today we all had haircuts at our house by our sister-in-law. At two and a half years old, Kendyl had her very first haircut. It was a little difficult to keep her still, but she sat on my lap while watching the TV show *Fancy Nancy*. Until today, her hair was quite uneven, but we had always been more worried about internal things that we did not think much about her hair. Both girls looked so cute and Alyx described it best as, "We are all fancy now."

July 2018

I was making dinner one night when I got a call from Make-A-Wish letting us know that Kendyl's wish had been granted and we would be going to Disney World. As exciting as it should have been, I burst into tears and told them I was grateful but that I couldn't think about it right now. I explained that she wasn't doing well and might even need another transplant. They were sad to hear the news but understanding. As I hung up the phone, I couldn't believe how much things had changed in such a short period. I even wondered if we would ever be taking this trip at all or if we might lose our baby girl. I couldn't help but think how sad it would be for her to be so close to having the trip of a lifetime and then never getting to experience it.

August 3, 2018

It was another long appointment day. We had early morning labs close to home and then drove to the further hospital to meet with the liver team.

We were a little relieved that Kendyl's ammonia level had come down to 116. It was still too high, but better than the last time we checked. Her weight had been the same at the past two appointments, so the team made more changes to her diet in hopes to keep her growing, without having too much protein. We were also waiting to see if our insurance would cover a special medication that might help bring the ammonia down. This was very expensive medicine. The doctors were not sure it would work but if it did, it could buy her some time before surgery. They were concerned that the level was not coming down and it could potentially cause brain damage if it stayed this high for too long.

They were evaluating what would be best for Kendyl and balancing the risks and benefits of every option. At this point, they thought that a surgery might be best, and it could take place as early as this month but would most likely happen in September. The procedure would try to force more blood flow through the liver, which would lower the ammonia. Her doctor mentioned that if it did not go as planned, she could need a second transplant and to be prepared in case it went that way. Although it was hard to face this possibility, we were relieved to know that the waiting list was not as long as it used to be (because of our amazing surgeon) and they were now able to do more transplants with living donors.

The team also wondered if her issues with aspiration and swallowing had been caused by the high ammonia. They feared that developmental delays were making it worse. The clinic had given us a lot of instructions to watch her closely for continued clumsiness, sleepiness, or anything else that seemed different about her development. It was hard as a parent to wonder each time she fell or was fussy if it was "normal" or if it might be the ammonia affecting her. It was so hard to watch our little one still going through so much in her young life. She was not even three years old yet!

August 4, 2018

We had a big day planned that we had been looking forward to. We were going to a picnic with people from the liver clinic, hang out as a family at Scheels (a sports store with fun activities as well, such as a Ferris wheel, bowling alleys, and more), and then have Kendyl participate in the Transplant Games that night. It was fun to see other transplant kids and their families at the picnic. We took a picture of all the kids who had received transplants. It was humbling to look at all those children and know that every single one of them had been saved because of an organ donor. For the most part, the kids looked happy and healthy, and you would never know about their conditions. When people asked how Kendyl was doing, I explained that she was doing OK but that she had some complications and would be having another surgery soon. Watching her with the other kids, she seemed to look sicker than some of them and I felt it was a glimpse of what was coming. I noticed she had a hard time with the heat, and by the time it was over she was done for the day, so we headed home. I was sad we missed the closing ceremonies (especially after seeing the pictures later) but I knew it was best for Kendyl. She was just exhausted.

Be grateful for the plans and activities that do happen.

August 8, 2018

After another long day with an ENT appointment, I really wanted to relax that night but felt the urge to donate blood again because it had been a little while. I looked for locations near me and there happened to be one around our area. We went as a family and Zach and I were both able to donate. The girls were crazy and running around but it was also special for them to be there. We were happy that they saw their parents doing something they felt was important.

August 11, 2018

If you want to feel out of place, go to a special couple's meeting by yourself. Zach and I had planned to attend a unique church meeting for couples married 10 years or less, but Kendyl's care had been a little difficult with her new medication and we did not want to leave her with anyone. The speaker, Ronald A. Rasband, shared many wonderful thoughts but the message I heard and felt the most was that we would be truly blessed for attending. I was touched that God knew it was hard for me to get to that meeting, especially by myself, and that it would have been a lot easier to skip the meeting. He knew I had a good excuse to stay home but that I made the effort to be there.

August 2018

Over the last few weeks, we had tried many medications to bring Kendyl's ammonia level down. We even went through major hoops with our insurance company to try to get the expensive medication covered, which we were so grateful for. However, none of them worked and we saw her level climb and affect her more and more. While most people didn't notice, as her mom and being with her all day, I could tell she was going downhill. She was speaking slower, using fewer words and seemed to have a harder time putting them together. She also continued to have more problems swallowing, choking, aspirating, and falling. I also noticed she had a rash on her cheeks and her gums were really swollen. It was heartbreaking to watch her and see such a difference, knowing she wasn't as healthy as she had been.

August 14, 2018

Kendyl had early morning labs, again, and her results came back with some concerns, such as low potassium, and still had high ammonia. She had been throwing up more and was not tolerating her special medication. When the team got the lab results, they decided to get her admitted so they could watch her closely. Her doctor also told us that they wanted to list Kendyl again for a second transplant just in case she needed it. I understood it was just a precaution and agreed to have her listed. It was better to have everything ready just in case there was an emergency, yet I could not believe we were experiencing it all again. We even met with the transplant coordinators again to go over what to expect with a transplant. As I listened to them, it made me realize just how much we had been through and what I had already forgotten. It was heartbreaking and exhausting to hear what we might have ahead us and I wondered if we had the strength to do it all again.

Since being admitted, Kendyl had lots of blood work, a GI study, echo, and an X-ray, while I continued to have transplant-education meetings. They were hoping to have everything done over a few days so she would be officially listed for the surgery scheduled on the 21st. Listing her now was in case something went wrong during surgery and turned into a worst-case scenario. I was grateful they were being cautious, but it was still hard to face.

Zach and I really felt that she needed the surgery, and we were glad it was happening soon since the ammonia continued to be a problem. We did not want her to have brain damage and hoped some of her swallowing issues would also get better. It was hard to process all my feelings. When I thought about it, my heart would ache, and my stomach would hurt. I never pictured going through a transplant again after just two years.

I will never forget how incredibly strong Kendyl was. Even while going through everything in the hospital and a high ammonia level of 126, she was still full of energy. The team kept expecting her to sleep a lot but that was not the case. Although she was a little clumsy walking because of her balance, she was still walking up and down the halls pushing a little baby doll in a stroller. I hoped that she had it in her to keep fighting and to, once again, pull through another major surgery.

Although the surgery was scheduled, the surgeon was open and straightforward with us. He wasn't sure it would be a success and told us there was a 25% chance Kendyl might not make it out of the operating room. The liver doctor reassured us that she had complete confidence. There were many phone calls and text messages back and forth between the team to discuss the risks.

We appreciated their transparency and concerns, but it was sometimes overwhelming.

August 18, 2018

The surgery was coming up in a few days but due to the uneasy feelings, the surgeon suggested a meeting to discuss it together. We drove to the hospital and met him and one of his students in the eating area of the front lobby. We were able to ask any questions and look at books and research that had been studied for cases similar to Kendyl's. Being a very busy doctor and surgeon, we were surprised that he spent over two hours with us (yes, he is that amazing), especially on a Saturday afternoon! It was something that I will truly never forget. I don't know how we had the good fortune to have the best liver doctor and the best surgeon. They truly cared and this was clearly shown through their actions.

After this meeting, we decided to go forward with the surgery. We let our family know, once again, that Kendyl would be having major surgery. At one point, we had told them that she would have it, later announced that it wouldn't happen, and once again it was a go. Even though we were still nervous about the surgery we confirmed the details. The procedure, estimated to be about six hours, would be happening the upcoming Tuesday and require a 7–10-day hospital stay. It was a week full of emotions, but we moved forward with faith.

August 20, 2018

We were settled in the hospital for the night so we could have her all prepped for the early morning surgery. I was happy that she was able to come home for a few days between her previous stay the week before and now being admitted again. She had been so fun and cute, and I loved the one-on-one time we got to spend together. Although I was nervous about the following day, I also felt so grateful for many people who had called, texted, brought treats, given hugs, posted on social media, came to visit, and for all the many prayers. I could truly feel them, and it meant so much.

I was grateful for Kendyl's amazing team and reassured that she was officially listed on the transplant list in case there was a major complication. I truly knew that the team cared about our little girl and that meant so much.

I tried to go to sleep but was feeling nervous, I wrote in my journal,

> *"Tomorrow my little, but tough, girl takes on another major surgery, fourth major surgery and only 2-years-old. It has been a crazy and stressful week. I heard heartbreaking statistics, words I hoped I would never hear from her doctors, held her down for too many pokes, IVs, and tests to even count. The surgery was scheduled last week but then for a day or two we debated whether it was the right thing and had to make the decision to go forward, knowing that they might not be able to fix her high ammonia issue. We are not sure what will happen tomorrow, but we know it is the right decision and we hope it will go as well as possible and delay another transplant for a long time. It is incredibly hard to watch your little one go through SO much. I would take any of it away if I could. Keep on fighting Kendyl Rose. You are so very loved."*

August 21, 2018

Zach came to the hospital early and stayed with us as we got Kendyl all prepped and ready. We were in a waiting area when somehow my mom joined us. I am still not sure how because I thought we were back in the operating prep area but somehow, someway, she was there and was grateful to see Kendyl before she went into the operating room. We signed multiple papers to give permission to the surgeon to take pictures, videos, and to provide training to other surgeons and doctors since it was the first time this type of procedure had been done at the hospital. We were grateful we could help by signing papers and allowing others to learn from her case to help other kids in the future. As we gave Kendyl to the team before the procedure, my mom told the surgeon that we had been praying for him. He responded with something like, "Thank you. I am just an instrument. We are a team." He also mentioned after that he appreciated the prayers. His response made us all cry, but we once again were comforted to know that Kendyl was in good hands.

We had family come down and stay with us in the waiting room, once again. We all came together wearing our new and updated "Kendyl Strong" shirts we had designed for the surgery. We tried to stay positive as we sat again waiting, hoping, praying, and welcomed each update we received through the hospital phone.

I will never forget seeing Dr. R's face when he had completed the surgery. He was sweaty and looked exhausted, which was something I never expected. I worried that maybe it was bad news with how he looked. However, as he came to the waiting room to see our family who had been waiting with us, he said the surgery went well and exactly how we had hoped and better than he could have imagined. He mentioned that she was stable the whole time and only received a small amount of blood at the end. He described in detail that he was able to take the major blood vessel that her body had created on its own, which was stealing blood flow from the liver, and put it where the original Rex Bypass was placed the previous year. The blood flow looked great so far and we hoped it would continue (especially the next 24–48 hours when it was most critical). Dr. R. believed that her body created the vessel shortly after transplant and it was "beautiful" and open and because her body created it on its own, it was the best-case scenario. He also showed us a picture and it looked beautiful! It was exactly what we had hoped and prayed would happen. We had prayed for a miracle, and we received it.

We were anxious to see her and were so relieved to see how peaceful she looked after. Even with all the tubes she looked great and again we never saw her on a breathing machine. We hoped to be able to get some rest and see her the next morning. Our hearts were so full, and we were beyond grateful for the news and prayers we felt that day.

It was interesting to look back and think about all the frustrations I had for months with the blood vessel that was stealing blood flow. A few weeks before the surgery they did one last CT scan to get a clear picture of what her body looked like inside and even I could see how big the blood vessel was and usually I couldn't read any CT scans. I just kept wondering why her body had to create it, why it was stealing the blood flow, and why it felt so unfair. It turned out to be the biggest blessing.

Sometimes the very thing you are complaining about is exactly what you need.

August 22, 2018

Kendyl Rose was doing amazing! Her ultrasound looked good, and her ammonia was down to 61. It had dropped by 50% in only 24 hours. The highlight of the day for me was two sessions of holding and snuggling her. She had been a little shaky and in pain a little bit, but overall, she had tolerated sips of water (her favorite), no throw ups (or gags) and even sat up on her own and tried to get down from her bed. She was getting back to herself today with her sayings such as "oh my gosh" and "stop it" and "not again" and also said, "I love you Mommy. I love you Daddy." It was the sweetest. She also said out of the blue, "I feel better." It was heartbreaking and joyful all at the same time. She was still in the PICU but if she continued to do well, she would be moved to her normal floor the following day. My heart was so grateful. I could not believe the discussions Zach and I were having the week previously with fear and tears compared to how she was doing today. We were seeing years of prayers being answered and it was a miracle.

August 23, 2018

She was walking within two days after having a major surgery. Even the IVs in both her feet were not going to stop her. Her ultrasound looked beautiful again and her ammonia was normal at 43. I could hardly believe it was that low and had changed so quickly. She had a few issues with throwing up, low potassium, very low magnesium, and needing some blood. It was these setbacks that kept her in the PICU instead of the regular floor as planned. However, we did get to switch to a nicer room that had some windows and a beautiful view. She looked great and later in the afternoon she finally fell into a deep sleep for the first time in days. God is good.

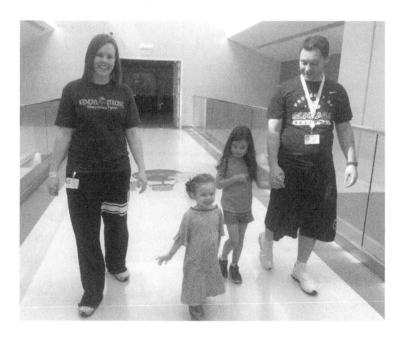

August 24, 2018

I was able to give our amazing surgeon a "Kendyl Strong" shirt that matched ours. I was feeling so incredibly grateful for him. He had now performed two major surgeries on our little girl. Both times I had been so impressed with his knowledge, experience, kindness, concern, and care. Each time he came to check on Kendyl he called her princess, and you could feel he truly cared about her. It was hard to express how grateful we were that he was there. When I first met him, two years previously, shortly after the transplant, I had no idea at the moment how appreciative our family would be for him. Without his transfer to our children's hospital, we would have had to go to Chicago for the last two surgeries since he was uniquely qualified to perform them. I can't even imagine how hard that would have been.

Having trust in your medical doctors and surgeons is so important.

August 25, 2018

There were so many emotions I was feeling. In my journal I wrote:

"Little one. I'm sorry I ever doubted you. I'm sorry I thought that the worst might happen and your time with us would be short. I know things can change quickly but right now I can hardly believe how well you are doing. It is an absolute miracle! If someone had told me how well the surgery would go, I wouldn't have believed it. However, it would have saved a lot of heartache and tears. You have always been small, but you are definitely fierce and that is why you are still with us. I can't even begin to express how much you have taught me. But today, you have reminded me to never give up. Even when things are really hard, you never know what miracles are right around the corner."

August 26, 2018

Alyx came to visit and the first thing she said to Kendyl was "Hi Sister. It's me. Do you remember me?" It was a wonderful day being together as a family for a few hours. The girls had been apart for a long week and to see them together was wonderful. I was also able to attend both church meetings at the hospital. I met some amazing sisters today and their stories were heartbreaking, but I also saw so much strength in each of them. I was humbled to realize that although we had been through a lot, it could have been much worse. We have been incredibly blessed. That night, Zach stayed with Kendyl, and I took Alyx home.

August 27, 2018

After spending the night at home in my own bed, Alyx and I had some fun quality time in the morning before her first day of kindergarten. I didn't think I would cry but I was a mess after dropping her off. I was excited for her but knew I would miss having her home with me. It felt scary to send her off into the world even though I knew it was a part of life.

I was excited to see her after her first day, but it broke my heart that she didn't have a good day. I was grateful to be there to pick her up and hear about it. I hoped with all my heart the next day would be better.

After I got Alyx home and cheered her up, I rushed back to the hospital and switched with Zach. I was grateful that he had been willing to stay with Kendyl and made it possible for me to have some time with Alyx. I appreciated taking her on her first school day and being there to hug her when she felt sad. I was now happy to be back with our little warrior. It was not easy to switch our time as the hospital was about an hour away, but it was always worth it.

Zach was going back to work the next day after taking some time off for the surgery. As much as I wished the time could have been spent on a family trip or something fun, I was grateful for the help. Kendyl continued to do well! She was happy (as long as no doctors or nurses were in the room) and looked the best she ever had in her life. She would be having a CT scan the next morning to make sure everything from the surgery was still looking well, and then she would probably be coming home the next day.

August 28, 2018

Our little miracle girl came back home after spending only seven days in the hospital. It was fun to put her in a "Kendyl Strong" shirt for the first time. I could hardly believe how great and big (all of a sudden) she now looked. It was the first time that a stay didn't go beyond what they said it would be, which was 7–10 days. Usually, we were way past it, but not this time. It was crazy to think that last week she was having major surgery and we were unsure if it would be successful. The last two nights were rough. Every time someone came in her room, day or night, she would scream as she thought they were going to poke her. However, the second she got home she was happy and back to drinking her water, which she loved.

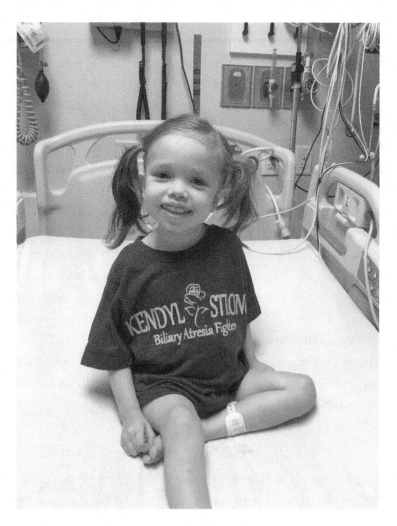

September 4, 2018

Kendyl had a liver clinic appointment today with both her doctor and surgeon. Her lab results were better than ever, and her ammonia was still normal. Everything looked so great that they felt confident they could stop checking it unless they had a concern. It was fun for them to see her and hear about the changes I had seen in the past two weeks. I noticed that she looked healthy, with no bruising, and the rashes on her face and arms were gone. She was eating and drinking well, and she was talking in longer and more complete sentences. Her gums were not swollen anymore, and she was not throwing up. Kendyl looked and seemed like a completely different little girl, much happier and calmer. It had been an amazing transformation with changes that both the surgeon, doctor, and us were not even expecting. We knew things could change quickly with her but at this moment, it felt like we had finally beaten the liver disease.

September 6, 2018

I had to give Kendyl a Lovenox injection shot in her thigh at 7:30 every morning and evening. This was by far the worst post-surgery care we ever had to give. Even though I knew she needed this blood thinner to keep the blood moving through the recently placed vessel and liver, it didn't make it easy. She always knew when it was coming so it would require both Zach and me to do it. She would fight hard to try to get away, crying and screaming, "Mommy, no!" It was heartbreaking and I dreaded it every single time.

It was a humbling experience, though. It caused me to frequently think about hard times and my relationship with God. When I know something is coming, even though it might be good for me, I sometimes kick and scream too because I don't understand why it's happening. The same was true with Kendyl. She did not understand why I had to poke her. All she knew was that it hurt.

God is aware of us and knows what is best for us. It is still hard, it still hurts, it might not make sense, and no matter how much we try to figure it out, we might yet not understand or see the whole picture at that time.

September 12, 2018

We were hanging out as a family after dinner when I got a call from Kendyl's surgeon. He told us that both her labs and ultrasound looked fantastic and that it was safe to stop her blood thinner shot. Everything was normal! Liver enzymes, electrolytes, ammonia, platelets, and everything else looked great. My sister had just happened to record the last Lovenox shot the night before to show Kendyl how brave she was. It melted my heart to hear Alyx ask if she could have the shot instead of her young sister.

The surgery was the biggest miracle, and I still could hardly believe it. It was surprising to see how well she was doing, especially considering that she was listed for a second transplant and now everything seemed to be "fixed!" My heart was so full.

For years, I kept remembering the prayer given in 2016 for Kendyl to "be healed quicker than anticipated." I clung to that every time she faced surgeries, such as the transplant in 2016, the Rex Bypass in 2017, and the Rex Bypass Revision in 2018. Two years later, after a transplant, two major surgeries, countless pokes, tears, and heartbreak, that prayer had finally been answered. It had happened, although not when I had pictured or would have liked it to happen.

September 14, 2018

I was able to donate Kendyl's special (and expensive) formula to a foundation for kids. This was the formula fed through her tube to try to lower her ammonia before surgery. I was grateful that she no longer needed it and happy that we could donate it to help others who might. While driving to deliver the formula, I just kept thinking about how amazing it is to know that so many foundations are there to help many people in need. When Kendyl was first diagnosed, I was impressed to learn about different programs and foundations I did not even know existed.

September 22, 2018

I felt like my heart might burst from joy. We were at Lagoon, a theme park near our house, and it felt like a dream come true to be there as a family. The girls had a blast, and it was so much fun watching them ride together and be there for each other. It was a little hard for me not to think of all the germs around us, but it was so worth it. There were many moments when I had to work hard to keep the happy tears in. I was hoping this was just the beginning of making fun memories and catching up for the past three years.

September 30, 2018

We were at church as a family. During the first meeting, known as the sacrament meeting, the congregation is given a small piece of bread and a small cup of water. It is very sacred. This time, Kendyl ate her whole piece of bread. It was a small piece but still a big moment that was very special to me. When I realized my thoughts had wandered, I had a sweet feeling that God knew how big that was for Kendyl and that He celebrated that win with me.

October 4, 2018

Kendyl had a big day of doctor appointments to see her liver team and a kidney doctor. We received so much good news. Her labs looked normal, and they decided to stop four medications: potassium, iron, amlodipine (a blood pressure med), and prednisolone (a steroid). It totally took me by surprise as I did not expect them to take her off the steroid any time soon. In fact, I actually never thought we would see that day. Her blood pressure was too low today (it was usually always high) so we hoped that dropping Amlodipine would bring the blood pressure back to normal. I was told to have her blood pressure checked with her pediatrician the following week but other than that, she was not scheduled for any labs or doctor visits for a whole month.

October 9, 2018

My phone rang and it was the liver clinic. I went into my bedroom so that I could hear well. I was told that because of the success of Kendyl's surgery, she would be taken off the transplant list. I immediately started crying as my heart was so full of gratitude. Reflecting about everything that had happened over the past several weeks, I could not believe where we were now. I couldn't help but think back to the time when we had wondered about going through with the surgery. We initially decided against it as it seemed scary and unlikely to go well. I was so deeply grateful that we went through with it.

November 2, 2018

After having a month off, Kendyl met with her liver team and her labs continued to look good. They were pleased with how well she was doing and that she was finally thriving! She was scheduled for a CT scan, which was standard after a big surgery, but they were confident that everything would be fine.

It was good news that Dr. B. did not feel the need to see Kendyl again for two months. I could hardly believe that her next appointment wouldn't be until after Christmas. She had seen this doctor at least once a month since we had moved back to Utah in February of 2016. The doctor also mentioned that she thought Kendyl would be off her feeding tube by the time she went to kindergarten. This was hard to believe but I hoped with all my heart that it would be true.

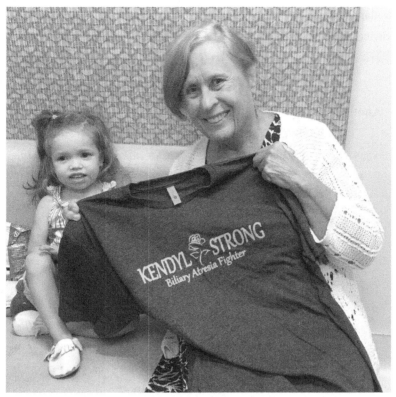

Kendyl and Dr. B.

November 12, 2018

Kendyl had the CT scan to look at the blood flow into her liver. She did great and the only tears came when inserting the IV and when taking it out. Since she was talking more, it was quite entertaining watching her come out of anesthesia. My favorite was when she asked if I was her mommy and when I answered yes, she said in a very slow voice, "You are my best friend." It was a precious moment.

After returning home, we decided to go Christmas shopping as a family. We figured it was a good way to keep Kendyl safe in her stroller as she was still a little tipsy from the medication given for the scan. That day felt normal and manageable. At this point I was trying to imagine our lives with less "liver-world" stuff. It was such a difference having standard check-ups, scans, and labs. For the first time ever, I was not worried about the results of her labs and tests.

November 13, 2018

Another journal entry:

"I waited so long for you to grow. It seems so sad when babies grow so fast, until you have one that doesn't and wears the same clothes for over a year at a time when they should be going through clothes like crazy. It felt like you were a newborn FOREVER with the amount of care you needed, and now I find myself missing my "baby" so much. Your toddler stage seemed short and now it feels you are just a little girl. I find myself wanting to hold you more than ever, wanting to feed you since I couldn't nurse you long and once you felt like eating you wanted to eat on your own and I never got that opportunity to feed you. In some ways I missed out on a lot of normal moments and milestones. I often feel my newborn baby stage was taken from me. Between my severe post-partum depression with Alyx and your diagnosis, I feel I got a little cheated. But I wouldn't trade you or your sister for anything. Some moments? Yes. (Most likely when you are fighting.) But overall, I just love you both to pieces and want to do the best I can for you both as your mom. My heart might hurt sometimes for our "lost time" or for a "normal baby experience" but it has taught me to really appreciate all the moments and make the best of each phase of life. It has also taught me that whatever stage you are in, good or bad, it won't last forever. Don't look too far in the future, or too far in the past. Focus on the moments you have right now."

December 2018

It was a normal day. We didn't go anywhere or do anything big. But we sang Christmas songs, laughed, danced and were happy. As a mom, I often feel that I don't plan enough big adventures, or do enough crafts and things like that, but that is not what life is about. You don't have to do something big and grand to have a good day.

December 12, 2018

We attended a Christmas Party with the liver team and the girls had so much fun. They had fun activities for the kids, such as cookie decorating, blow up balloons, and even Santa made a visit. My favorite part was seeing so many kids of all ages running around and acting like kids, and not knowing which were "transplant kiddos" and which were siblings. It was wonderful! Observing them, I kept thinking of all the donors who had saved so many lives.

> The ripple effect of organ donation is huge. It does not only affect the donor family and participants; it affects extended families and many people around them.

December 22, 2018

It was the first year that Kendyl came with us to deliver books to the hospital to give as gifts, which was a big deal for us. We were usually too worried about germs to bring her. I was deeply grateful to see her run up and down the hall. Seeing kiddos walking the halls while hooked to machines was a reminder of a time that was still fresh in our memories.

End of 2018

It was another year with many ups and downs, but it was mostly filled with miracles. I felt so appreciative for where we were, especially considering where we had been. During the year, there were many times when I was grateful just watching Kendyl with the clothes that Alyx used to wear. I had often wondered if I would ever see it. This also made me realize how young and small Alyx was when we moved. She still talked about friends that she left behind. They had both been through a lot during that crazy time. The journey wasn't over, but at this time, I felt incredibly grateful, happy, and proud of where we were.

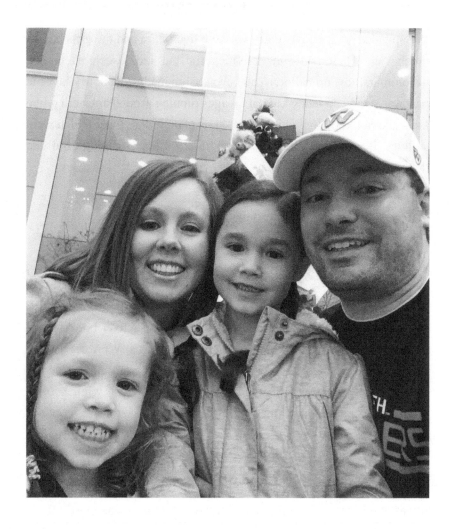

Chapter 5
LiveReal
2019

January 1, 2019

Instead of giving sibling gifts for Christmas, my family thought it would be fun to provide a meal at the Ronald McDonald Room at Primary Children's Hospital. We had hoped to serve dinner during the Christmas season, but it was booked for the entire month of December. We were initially disappointed that the earliest day available was January 1st, but it turned out to be a perfect day.

I went to the hospital with my parents to carry in the food and start preparing. An hour later, the rest of the family joined us, and we served food for everyone. It felt different but so good to be on the other side of the table. I had been there for several meals in the past, often with a heavy heart and tired eyes, and always felt so grateful for a fresh and free meal. I remember being there while wondering if my daughter would be OK and the sadness that was felt with each new challenge and obstacle. We were so grateful for the opportunity to serve. Many people thanked us and expressed their gratitude. I understood their situation and I knew they meant it. As I watched my girls playing in the room that day, my heart was so full. Seeing Kendyl running around, eating snacks and being a crazy and thriving girl was amazing. When someone asked about the "Kendyl Strong" shirts we were wearing, we would point to our miracle girl and share a little bit about her story. My heart hurt when some people shared their stories. It was interesting how hearing someone else's story made me feel instantly connected. A small act of service and time spent with family was such a wonderful way to start the new year. I hope to always be able to create strong memories with our girls and to give back to those in need. Even when helping in small ways, it makes a big difference to those who receive it.

> Service can be fun. Find others to serve with. Not only will it help those you serve but you will feel better too.

January 25, 2019

This was a magical night! The girls had received beautiful dresses from Make-a-Wish a few days prior and this was the night we got to put those on our own little princesses. We told the girls that we were going to a special party.

Our wish granters greeted us as we arrived, along with some of our family. A few minutes later we were greeted by princesses Anna, Elsa, Rapunzel, and Elena. The girls' faces were full of joy. They enjoyed having snacks with the princesses and stared at them and their pretty dresses as they danced around the room.

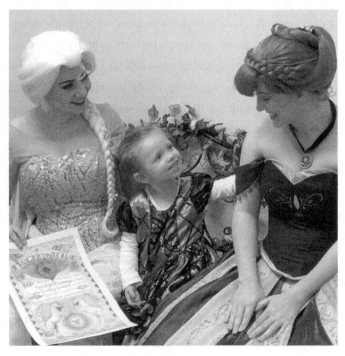

Although the girls would have been happy that night just spending time with the princesses, that wasn't the big surprise. They sat Kendyl down on a chair in the middle and read a beautiful scroll saying her wish had been granted and she would be going to Disney World. I couldn't hold in the tears. We felt excited and relieved to know that we could now talk about the trip without spoiling the surprise since we were scheduled to leave in less than two weeks. She was also given a cute banner to take home for counting down the days. It was a night full of smiles and happy tears.

February 5–11, 2019

A few days before our trip to Disney World our wish grantors came to our home with the itinerary, shirts and bags for all, a backpack for Kendyl and activities for the girls to do on the plane. They even arranged to have the feeding and medical supplies shipped ahead of us so we wouldn't have to carry so much in our luggage. It was so well organized and thoughtful; it made us even more excited for the trip.

When the big day arrived, my mom took us to the airport, and we flew from Utah to Dallas and then on to Florida. We arrived several hours later and were greeted by a volunteer from Give Kids the World (GKTW) which is a special nonprofit resort in Kissimmee, Florida for children with critical illnesses and their families. The volunteer had a sign that said, "Welcome Kendyl" and was holding a Shimmer and Shine balloon. We picked up the vehicle they had rented for us (a red van that the girls' thought was so cool), including car seats, and made our way to GKTW. We had a little issue with our luggage, but the airport staff located the missing bag and brought it later that night.

We stayed for a week in our purple house #104 and chose to visit Hollywood Studios, Universal Studios, Bibbiddi Bobbidi Boutique, Epcot, and Magic Kingdom. The girls loved the rides, especially Frozen at Epcot, and meeting all the princesses and characters. They also loved getting them to sign their signature books. It was something that daddy knew nothing about, so the girls showed him how it's done. Their favorite thing was our special genie pass that allowed us to skip the lines for rides and meeting characters. I was amazed by the arrangements that were available to us, such as a special area we had one night to watch the fireworks at Magic Kingdom. It was incredible to see the joy on Kendyl's face after all she had been through and to experience it as a family.

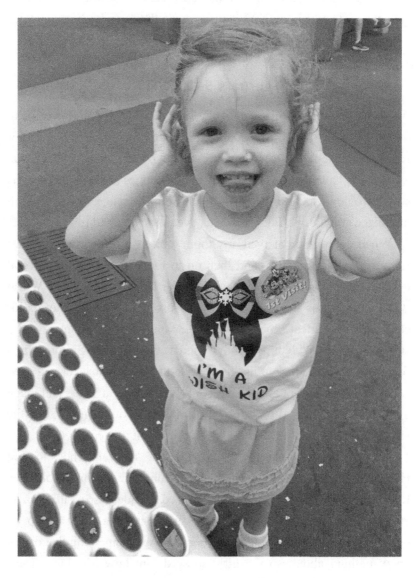

As amazing as the theme parks were, GKTW was also a highlight of the trip. The village is mostly operated by volunteers who give a lot of their time to serve. It was impressive to watch those who happily cared for us during our stay. Each morning we ate breakfast at GKTW and there were a lot of options, including ice cream at any meal (even breakfast). Each day, the girls would be given special gifts to take home. After being at the park all day, we would come back every night to eat dinner at GKTW and then attend activities at the village. That included Christmas with Santa, Candy Land game night, bunny tuck ins and more. We were also able to watch the movie Coco in the GKTW movie theater and Kendyl was given a special star to hang up in a special room filled with stars by other Make-a-Wish kiddos.

It was the most magical week! Honestly, it was a little overwhelming and I found myself feeling guilty at times. However, I kept reminding myself of what we had been through and tried to express thanks to everyone around us. Although we couldn't have afforded to go at that time, we also would not have dared to go with Kendyl's care and the supplies she needed. The parks and GKTW definitely know how to care for those with illnesses.

The last night of the trip Zach and I decided it would be fun to watch a movie together after the girls went to bed. I called the office and innocently asked if they had adult movies … there was a long awkward pause and she said they only had kid movies. I got off the phone and Zach was laughing and shaking his head. I couldn't figure out why. He then asked me if I knew what adult movies were. I replied that they were PG-13 like my favorite movie *The Proposal*. Nope, apparently it meant something else. It was a funny moment and something we still laugh about today.

Even though the trip was a few years ago, we still talk about it often and recall the memories that were made that week. It was so good for our family and really brought us together as we experienced a trip filled with joy. I hope to be able to give back as a GKTW volunteer when the girls are older. We look forward to serving there together as a family.

If I could give anyone any advice about a similar trip (or any trip), it would be to make a plan while remaining flexible with it. I had plans for each day based on what activities were going on at both GKTW and the various Disney parks, and also considered the weather. However, each day we were flexible too. We had absolutely no regrets about our once-in-a-lifetime trip, which is exactly how it should be.

Make-a-Wish is an incredible organization, and I would strongly encourage donating to support it, if you are able. You can help kids receive wishes they will remember forever.

February 2019

Journal entry:

> *"I love the bond that my girls share. It truly melts my heart. I always pictured having more than two kids, but after Kendyl and her journey our plans changed. When I see how close my girls are, it makes me feel it might be OK that way. Lately Alyx had been telling Zach and I that if something happened to us, she would take care of her sister. She specifically mentioned she would give Kendyl her meds and take her to Disneyland. Hopefully, Zach and I will be around for a while, but I do hope these two will always stay friends, always give hugs, and always be there for each other."*

April 10, 2019

It was an awful morning with labs. We went to the nearby hospital where we had been going recently. They poked Kendyl three times and they still weren't able to get enough blood. That made it necessary to travel to the more distant one the following day. I felt so bad for our little warrior. After this experience we never went back to that hospital for labs, even though it was a lot closer. It was worth the longer drive to have a better lab experience. Our girl was hard to poke so it was just a better option for us. She looked small, but she was stronger than she appeared to be. I was grateful that the next day we got through the labs with more ease and tried to make up for the traumatic experiences with doughnuts.

April 18, 2019

We had big news in our house. Our miracle girl was now potty trained. It was something I was proud of, and grateful for as well. It wasn't about buying diapers; it was about knowing that we had crossed this major milestone. It was another one that I wondered if we would ever reach. I even took a picture with her new Shimmer and Shine panties, below her scarred belly, with her potty chart.

June 5, 2019

After everything Kendyl had been through the previous fall, it was now time to take the swallow study. I was nervous about getting her to drink the pasty and chalky drink for the test, just like the first time. I did my best to stay calm and bribed her that if the test went well, I would take her to get a doughnut after. I hyped up the sprinkles, pink frosting and anything else I could think of.

The swallow study went well. She didn't drink much but enough so they could get some images. Her therapist was there and told us that she thought Kendyl was swallowing flawlessly. She told us to wait for the results, but she was very confident that she had passed with flying colors. A few days later the results confirmed her observations.

This was a huge step! We were so excited. This meant that she would no longer need thickened liquids. We had started at honey thick after her ammonia level went from very high, down to nectar thick. This result meant that we could now focus on getting her off the G-tube.

I'm sure there is research against this, and some would argue with me, but I think it's OK to bribe your kids. My belief is that those who don't agree simply haven't been in these situations. If a pink doughnut with sprinkles helps with a swallow study, I'm all for it. This doesn't happen often but for situations like this, it is absolutely worth it. Unless you've been in a similar situation, just trust me on this.

Summer of 2019

The girls took a dance class together during the summer. Since it was only for a few weeks, they were able to be in the same class. I'm not sure the instructors would agree, since the girls often didn't listen and would fight at times, but for me, having them in the same class was the best thing.

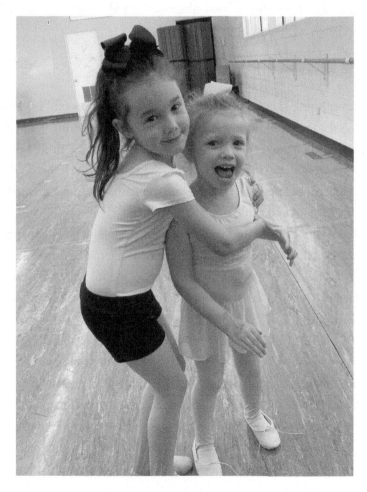

My journal entry described the experience as:

"I remember watching them one day in class with their cute pink leotards and ballet shoes. I realized, as I watched them, that these were the days I was dreaming of while I was pregnant with Kendyl. I dreamed of two girly girls, lots of hair, lots of pink and purple things in our home, and dance classes. I never dreamed or pictured liver disease, surgeries, medications, feeding tubes, organ donation, doctor appointments, labs, hospital stays and more. I am so glad I didn't know it at the time because I was already nervous to go from one child to two. I realized it had taken me years to have these moments that I had dreamed of. But it was worth the wait, and it made me enjoy it so much more. I felt my heart might burst as I watched them both dance in the same class in the same studio I danced at for years."

November 6, 2019

Kendyl had a tonsillectomy. Her tonsils were big, she was snoring at night, and we knew that with time, if she tested positive for Epstein-Barr Virus (EBV), she would need to get them out. We wondered if she would eat better, and also wanted to get them out while she still had her G-tube to be sure she would remain hydrated.

As we drove to the hospital in the dark, early that morning, she kept asking quietly, "Where are we going?" I didn't have the heart to tell her, and I also didn't want to get her upset before arriving. I found creative ways to change the subject and focus on something to look at on our drive.

We arrived and got her dressed and ready. When it was time, she got in a little wagon while watching her electronic tablet and a doctor pulled her into the operating room. It was so different than it had been in the past when I would hold her and put her in the arms of the doctor. This made me realize how much older she was.

The procedure was quick, but the report indicated that she struggled to fall asleep. It broke our hearts to wonder what she had been through without us being there. When it was time to see her, it was one of the saddest moments ever. She was crying, very upset and confused. It absolutely broke my heart. I had seen her with big incisions, lots of wires and more, but this moment sticks out as one of the hardest post-op times to see her. I was grateful when she was more awake, less confused, and happier.

We prepared ourselves for a few rough weeks after the procedure, but it was almost as if nothing had happened! There were two times when she said, "My throat feels weird," but that was all. She didn't even mention any pain. Once again, it reminded me how tough she was.

Throughout her life, I had felt that life was so unfair for her, and the situation seemed harder because she was a baby. I had convinced myself that it would have been easier on all of us if these issues had come up when she was older. However, after watching the small procedure of getting her tonsils removed, I realized what a blessing it was that she was a baby through all the rough years.

End of 2019

It was interesting that after Kendyl seemed to be "fixed" and thriving, I started having some very minor health challenges. I had sinus infections frequently, was sick more often, and had a lot more doctor appointments than I had ever had. Although it was annoying, I felt grateful that these small issues came after Kendyl was doing so well. I can't imagine what it would have been like to deal with these issues while caring for Kendyl so intently. It was such a blessing.

Chapter 6
LiveReal
2020

January 24, 2020

We were cleared for Kendyl to take her meds by mouth. This was a big step toward getting rid of the G-tube. The transition was making me nervous, but I felt it was time. I had been told to mix the medication with chocolate syrup or to have them filled with flavor at the pharmacy. However, I chose to give them the way they were and see what happened. The first time I gave her the meds orally, it was a little awkward and she wasn't quite sure about it. She described it as "spicy," which was hard for me to understand since I couldn't taste it. Since that first time, she has taken them like a champ. I am happy that I decided to give them by mouth the way they were, without extra sugar.

Sometimes it can be a blessing to not know what we are missing. I'm grateful that flavored meds exist. I'm sure this is a life-saving option for many parents dealing with sick kids. Since Kendyl doesn't know that option is available, and she doesn't make a fuss about it, the original option is better and easier for us.

February/March 2020

Life was really feeling "normal," and it felt amazing. Kendyl was taking all her medications by mouth and was no longer using the G-tube at night, which was so great. Zach and I used to do the rock-paper-scissor method to see who would prepare her formula, prime her tubing, and hook her up each night. It was so nice not having to worry about her feeds. It gave us more time to be alone at night after the girls were in bed.

Life was good! It felt like a worrisome chapter of our lives was coming to an end. We even planned to get season tickets to the Lagoon theme park in our area. It was a big moment when we realized that we felt comfortable taking Kendyl out of the house, and even to a germy place, but it was also exciting that we could afford it.

And then, the world shut down. The Covid-19 virus spread worldwide, and we found ourselves staying home again to keep Kendyl safe. This timing was really hard for us. For years, we had stayed home trying to keep her safe, and when we finally felt comfortable to do more, this virus made us nervous and kept us home. It really felt unfair as we had already lived this life for years. We were ready to live normally.

Just like everything in life, there was a split side. We could focus on being frustrated with our situation or we could focus on the fact that Kendyl wasn't in the hospital at a time when they were overburdened. We were grateful that she was thriving at home instead.

Another challenge for us was dealing with harsh judgment from others who didn't understand our situation. We didn't expect everyone to do what we were doing, but it hurt to have people ridicule us for doing what we felt was best for Kendyl and for our family.

No one knows your situation. Stay true to what you believe is right. It might be different from what the world is doing and that is OK.

April 2020

I was feeling disappointed and stuck. The world continued to shut down, so we remained home. I knew that I needed something that would keep me going. I was excited when I discovered an incredible mindset coach and mentor from the Proctor Gallagher Institute. I knew immediately that I had stumbled on someone who could help me. It was a big investment and felt like a scary move when the future was unknown, but I could not shake the feeling that I had to go forward and bet on myself.

This one decision affected my life in ways I could have never dreamed of. It was by far the best choice I made in 2020. After being coached for a few months, I was able to take on some leadership roles with my coach. It was an incredible experience to share the tools that I have learned with others. I really enjoy helping people feel their best, through simple health solutions and mindset tools, and facilitating change from the inside out.

There is a quote that says, "When the student is ready, the teacher appears." I believe this is true.

June 7, 2020

It was important for Kendyl to consume enough water to protect her kidneys (which was currently 45 oz/day). Although she had done this occasionally before, we decided it was time to make a firm decision to not use her feeding tube anymore.

Because of the focus I had on my mindset and the tools that I had learned from my mentor, I developed great confidence in myself and also in Kendyl's abilities. I knew that I could help her and believed that she could do it. From this day on, she drank her minimum goal every single day. Some days were easier than others, but we never looked back. This is not a typical story for most kids with G-tubes but it was for her. It felt like the investment in myself not only affected me but my whole family for the better.

A month or so later, the feeding therapist called to see Kendyl again (appointments had been on hold due to Covid). When I informed her that she was drinking all her fluids by mouth (which was the only thing keeping in her therapy), she was both shocked and excited. We never went back to therapy. It was such a great thing that she was able to graduate. Unfortunately, Kendyl never had the chance to say goodbye to her friend "Michelle."

August 2020

Another school year began. With the worldwide pandemic, we debated for months about what to do but decided that keeping Alyx at home was the best option to keep Kendyl safe. We knew it would be hard for her since she was a social girl and thrived at school. We also pulled Kendyl out of preschool. She was sad that she wouldn't be able to experience what her sister did, which was something she had been looking forward to. However, we knew these decisions were for the best.

Online learning was different than we thought it would be. The school was fantastic and did everything possible to help with our situation. Every day, Alyx would sign into Zoom for the entire school day, and she wore uniforms as if she was in the classroom. It was hard to have her home because she couldn't play with her sister. Keeping her focused on schoolwork was a real challenge.

We felt helpless as parents, and we were not quite sure what to do in this situation. We loved both of our girls and knew their needs were different and tried to do the best we could under these circumstances. Deciding to get some counseling allowed us talk through our situation and it really helped.

November 12, 2020

Our little miracle girl was tube free! Technically, she had been without it for about a week because it had fallen out. I had had a hard time getting it back in so they told us that we could leave it out. After a short outpatient procedure, the G-tube opening was now surgically closed. I hoped that it would heal well, since this added another scar to her little belly.

It was surreal to look back on our journey with a feeding tube, and to realize that we had reached this point. I had often wondered if we would ever reach this milestone. Kendyl had had a tube for most of her life, starting when she was only four months old. The first tube had been replaced with a longer-term G-tube when she was two years old, and it was now removed permanently three years later. Every type of feeding tube had been inconvenient, but they had saved her life. We didn't want that reality to get lost while celebrating that she was finally tube free.

A few thoughts from my journal:

> *"Kendyl Rose I am so proud of you all that you continue to teach me. I am sad I missed out on feeding you through the years with nursing, a bottle, and even with utensils. These were all things I didn't really get to do. However, I was able to witness a miracle. I was able to watch modern medicine and a feeding tube help you grow. I was able to witness two amazing feeding therapists who helped you on your journey and gave tips that I could have never thought of on my own. I was able to watch prayers be answered. I was able to watch you go from not eating or drinking anything to now eating everything (it feels like) and drinking your goal of 45 oz each day to keep your liver and kidneys happy. I've missed out on some normal things with you, but I've experienced and learned so much since you were born that have made me stronger. After all these years where you would usually be connected by some type of cord, and sometimes multiple at time (such as feeding tube, TPN, lipids, PICC line, etc.), you are free. I am grateful that all went well, and that daddy could be there too. What a happy day! I think six surgeries in five years is good for a long time and I know you will continue to thrive living life. You are the bravest, sweetest, and toughest girl I know. You truly are a miracle."*

The G-tube closure was the most minor of all Kendyl's surgeries and yet, it was a hard one for me emotionally. A few days before the surgery I was a wreck, and I could not quite figure out why. After reflecting about this, I eventually put it together. I was losing an identity that I had carried for over four years, a feeding tube momma. It was an identity that I thought I might have forever. I thought it would be easy for me to let go of this identity, and yet it took some time. There was a proud feeling of graduation in my heart, and yet a feeling of nervousness for what was next. Maybe a part of me felt like I wasn't needed as much.

The experience taught me a lot and I've often reflected on it and the growth that came along with it. After this experience, I knew it was time for me to chase some of my own dreams, such as writing this book.

There might be an identity that you are
holding on to that needs to be let go.

Chapter 7
LiveReal
2021

January 2021

When the new year started, we re-evaluated if it was time to send Alyx back to the classroom. She was struggling with e-learning and getting low scores on tests. It was getting worse over time, with some as low as 30%. We knew that going back to school would help her, but we still worried about the risk for her sister. After thinking and praying about it for a while, we decided it was now time. She went back to school and started to thrive again.

Being a parent is hard. It is especially challenging with multiple kids, even just two. It's difficult, at times, to balance what is best for both.

Fall of 2021

There were trials that I never thought I would experience. Trials that forced me to learn lessons I would not have learned any other way. Although they have been hard, I know without a doubt that the Lord was with me through them all. I also believe that each experience helped me to become stronger and prepared me for the next one. I am so grateful to know that we are not alone and with God's help, whatever hard times we go through won't be more than we can handle. I know that when we go through trials, we often begin to see most blessings and miracles.

Kendyl is absolutely thriving. This girl has the sweetest little heart and is always thinking of others. She has a fun personality and loves her sister. After living in and out of the hospital for years, it is an absolute miracle that she has not been back since the Rex-Bypass Revision in August of 2018. She is now down to a single anti-rejection medication that she takes morning and night.

Life is pretty good and almost normal, except a few minor things. Her suppressed immune system will keep her away from lakes and swimming pools to avoid infections that could destroy the liver. She needs to drink more fluids than most children. But, even with these small things, life is better than I ever dreamed it could be. Kendyl looks like a normal girl and for the most part she is. If you didn't know her and her story, you would never guess what she has been through. You can't see it today, but the experiences were real, and the trials and fears felt endless. We are all forever changed.

I know that not everyone will have such a happy story. Many will unfortunately lose their life to biliary atresia since there is no cure. Sadly, some will get too sick before receiving their gift of life through organ donation.

I hope that our family's journey will help you keep the faith that better days are ahead and trust that everything will be well. My intention was to provide hope and support for anyone going through similar experiences or hardship. One of my favorite quotes is, "Everyone is fighting a battle. Be kind." Don't judge those around you. You might never know what battles they are fighting or what they have been through that can't be seen.

Kendyl's journey, despite so many hard times, was full of miracles. May her courage be a source of inspiration to keep going when facing any challenge. Don't give up.

Chapter 8

LiveReal

Zach's Story

(This chapter is from Zach's perspective.)

December 11, 2015

In my third year of law school, I did not have any Friday classes so I would use those days to study what I had learned through the week and to prepare for Monday. I specifically chose this schedule so that I could maximize my time with my wife and our little girls. Little did I know, this would be the last normal Friday I would have for quite some time.

Samantha called me shortly after lunch and she was sad because Kendyl's doctor visit did not go as she had planned. It felt like she needed me, so I told her to come pick me up at school and that I was done studying for the week. I did not think this would be a big deal and initially thought that she might have been over-reacting, but sometimes a husband just needs to be there to support his wife.

After reassuring Samantha that everything was going to be all right and waiting for her to arrive, I spent a few minutes on Google to see what it had to say about bilirubin. I was initially relieved with the results since none of them indicated that it was a big deal (proving that a Google MD cannot replace the real kind).

We had plans to attend a Christmas Party that night but when Kendyl's doctor called with the results, our lives were really changed. We were told to immediately go to Sacred Heart Hospital in Spokane and that they would be expecting us. I began to realize that I was wrong to think this was not a big deal, but I was still not too worried that this would be a major hurdle. My thought was that she might be in the hospital for the weekend and while that would be inconvenient, everything would return to normal early the following week after her release.

The four of us immediately left for the hospital. We really did not know where we were supposed to go but I dropped off Sam and Kendyl at an entrance and went to park the car. As I carried Alyx inside, we somehow found the right spot and the four of us began waiting in a room, not sure what the future would hold for us.

The shock of this sudden change was something none of us could have foreseen. It was starting to be late and little Alyx, who was just a two-year-old, was behaving well, but a hospital room is not the most ideal place for them. After initial conversations with doctors, Samantha and I decided that it would be best for me to get Alyx home in her bed. I left kind of shell shocked. I was leaving my wife and daughter at the hospital that night and it felt surreal that so much could happen in so little time.

Before Alyx and I left the hospital, I sent a text message to two of my best friends. A thread that was usually filled with insults and talk about sports was now filled with messages of support and love. I still remember the drive home that night. I was trying to explain what was going on to Alyx and told her that things would be different for a little while, but we would all be together again in the same house one day.

Once we were home, I made dinner for Alyx and then got her to bed. I called Samantha for an update and tried my best to lift her spirits. It was important for me to be present and strong so she could lean on me, but that is often a difficult task. Anyone in a similar situation has probably felt the same way and that their support was inadequate. That night, when I went to bed, I was concerned about the road ahead for our little family, but I was glad that I had a partner like Samantha that I could rely on and work as a team with to overcome what was before us.

KASAI SURGERY — DECEMBER 17, 2015, and FINALS WEEK

Before sharing my perspective about the Kasai Surgery, I must give proper recognition to Gonzaga University and the administrators and law professors I worked with there. The staff at Gonzaga told me that they would allow me to push my finals to February so I could deal with the situation with Kendyl. Samantha and I discussed this option and while I appreciated the possibility, we ultimately decided that taking my finals as scheduled would be best.

Taking the finals in February, along with five other classes, would have been overwhelming. Although my preparation in the last week was not where I wanted it to be, I had studied all semester. If I took the finals as scheduled, I would have no studying or classes for three weeks until the final semester of law school would begin the second week of January.

My professors and the Dean of the Gonzaga Law School were great to work with. I would often get calls or e-mails to make sure that Kendyl was doing okay and that my family had everything that we needed. They also told me to make sure that my mind was clear during the tests. I truly appreciate that they took such great care of me and to also feel that they cared deeply about what was happening with my little girl.

My final exam was on the same day as the Kasai Surgery. The exam was scheduled to end at noon and our girl would be taken for surgery shortly thereafter. My professor knew that I was going to the hospital for the surgery right after the final. I will never forget when on my way out after the exam she said, "now go take care of that little girl and don't even think about school."

I was happy to get there in time to have a few moments with Sam and Kendyl before she was taken for her surgery. Time crawls when you wait for a child to come out of surgery. I barely remember what we did while she was in surgery, but I do recall speaking with the doctor afterward and being reassured that he felt it went okay.

It was a big relief to be done with school for three weeks so I could focus on taking care of my family and help Kendyl recover from the surgery. I never imagined myself spending so many hours in a hospital with a sick child, but this was my new reality. Although I was overwhelmed and tired at times, there were also many sweet moments that I still cherish.

DECEMBER 31, 2015

Kendyl was finally going to be discharged from the hospital. After 21 days, our family would be home together under one roof. Samantha and I had delayed our Christmas celebration until January 2nd (it was a fun and wonderful day).

I still remember the night when a nurse came over to show us how we would administer Kendyl's meds through the central line that went directly to her heart. I could not believe that it was going to be up to Samantha and me to administer IV meds to our daughter's heart without any help from a medical professional. The nurse told us that we would be fine, and while I tried to appear confident for my wife, deep down I thought there was no possible way that we would be able to do that.

After this training, I left to go pick up Alyx at a friend's home. I remember feeling completely overwhelmed on the drive back. I thought to myself this was way too much and worried that Kendyl was not going to receive the care she needed because Samantha and I were not capable to do what was expected from us.

Thankfully, we had so much help and support from many good friends and neighbors in the Spokane area. I am not sure how we will ever let them know how much their help truly meant to us.

Somehow, one day turned into two days and then a week and we gained more confidence to do things we would never have dreamed of doing. I still can't believe the feelings of depression and overwhelm were replaced with confidence and strength. Samantha and I would constantly say to each other to "keep grinding, we can be tough for one day." We continued to work together and to be supportive of one another. It is that teamwork that got us through the seemingly insurmountable obstacles in front of us.

When we started this medical journey, neither of us had any real knowledge or skills with anything related to first aid care. Now we can both confidently place a feeding tube, give IV meds through a PICC or a central line, place a G-tube to give meds or run feeds, just to name a few. It was a long and difficult process, but it was one made easier because I had a dedicated partner and we worked together to achieve a common goal.

SPOKANE'S MOST INELIGIBLE BACHELOR

In February 2016, we determined that the best course of action for Kendyl's care and for Samantha's support system was to have them move back home to Utah. They would be close to Primary Children's Hospital in Salt Lake City, while I finished my last semester of law school at Gonzaga. This was a difficult and wearisome time for our family, so we tried to do a FaceTime call every night to keep a strong connection to each other. I am grateful for the blessings of modern technology that enabled us to do that.

It was during this time that I would refer to myself as Spokane's Most Ineligible Bachelor. I was happy that Samantha had plenty of help back home. While I knew that a temporary separation was best for our family, even if it was harder on me, I was often depressed and felt alone.

As the days went by, I could feel myself becoming angrier and shorter tempered. I seemed to get more frustrated when people cut me off in traffic or if something didn't go as planned. This was all internal anger as I really was never close enough to anyone to say mean things. This separation was challenging me, and I just was not happy in life. I tried to put on a fake happy face when I would talk with my family so that they would not worry about me. My focus remained on Samantha and the girls.

I often joked with Samantha that the only good thing about our separation was that I could watch the NCAA Tournament and the NBA

Playoffs without my wife nagging me to do chores and little kiddos trying to divert my attention away from the TV. While I say this in a joking tone, the reality is that sports probably helped me to forget my problems and allowed me to let go of the anger I was feeling.

I was grateful that my professors and the administration at Gonzaga University were understanding of what I was going through. Law School is taught using the Socratic Method and students are expected to be prepared and knowledgeable about the topics to be discussed in class that day rather than the teacher giving a lecture. Teachers would often engage in a debate or conversation with many students, and this would all be done at random. Students had to be prepared to talk about all of the topics and potential counterpoints if they wanted to avoid being embarrassed in front of their peers. Since my professors were all aware of my situation, instead of calling on me at random they would often e-mail me a few days before and ask if I would be prepared to talk about a certain subject in class. I appreciated these efforts to spare me of potential public embarrassment, but I still wanted to be challenged and grow in my learning and understanding. This attention made me feel like the teachers and administrators at Gonzaga University really got involved in the lives of their students and that they truly cared.

After I finished my last final, I went to the Spokane Airport to pick up my parents and Samantha's father. My mom and my father-in-law went to our house and started packing our belongings while my dad and I went to play golf at the famous Coeur d'Alene course. (I hit a beautiful 7-iron to about 15 feet on the 14th hole island green. Unfortunately, I missed the birdie putt but tapped in for a par.)

The next day, my wife flew up to Spokane and surprised me because she wanted to be there when I walked with my graduating class. I was shocked to see her running toward me up our street after we had just finished loading up the U-Haul (typical of her to show up after the work is done, just kidding). Samantha and I went out to dinner that night and it was fun be together again after being apart for so long.

As I walked in the graduation ceremony the next day with a JD/MBA dual degree from Gonzaga University, I couldn't believe all the challenges the last year brought our way. I looked at my wife seated in the audience and felt so much gratitude for her and the support and guidance she brings to my life. Her influence has greatly shaped many of the choices I have made. I never could have done any of the major things I have done in life without her by my side. Over the last few months, there were many times when I felt that I could not go any further. She carried me and lifted me up to her high standard, even when I felt overwhelmed. There is no other person that I would have wanted by my side to go through these trials.

TAKING THE BAR AND FINDING A JOB

After graduating law school in May, I was not done studying, because the Bar Exam awaited in late July. In a way, it was just starting as I began to study intensively for the following two months. Under the circumstances, it was quite an undertaking to face this while helping Samantha raise our girls. Our main focus was keeping Kendyl alive and healthy enough to handle a transplant surgery.

While preparing for the Bar Exam, the stress of life was often overwhelming. The anxiety that I felt while trying to become the provider that my wife and girls deserved was a burden. I tried not to show this on the outside, but it was wearing on me. One of the most depressing feelings a man can have is of not doing an adequate job of providing for his family. It is a fear, or an embarrassment, that I am positive all men have, and I was no different. I probably put even more pressure on myself because of what was before me, and I felt that Samantha and my girls deserved so much.

Kendyl's health was declining rapidly, and the yellow jaundice color was spreading from her eyes, through her skin, and even showing in her dark hair. It was a gut-wrenching feeling to watch my little one slowly moving closer to death and there was very little I could do to stop it. Samantha and I did everything we could together for our girl, we did her meds, her feeds, and we were up at all hours of the night together, cleaning her bed and doing laundry when she would throw up. It was an incredibly draining time. We were overwhelmed and exhausted, but we were together and supported each other through these challenging times. There is no way we would have gotten through these trials on our own. This took unwavering efforts from both of us along with the steadfast support we received from our extended family. It was so much that this book could not contain it all.

After the Bar Exam, I began my search for a job. I had done some legal work while I was in my last year of law school and began to feel that perhaps law was not the field I was set on entering. I was open to any possibility, willing to explore opportunities. After many interviews and disappointments, I finally received an offer from a very respected institution. This has been such a huge blessing for me and my family. The despair and insecurity I felt as a husband and a father about providing for my wife and my girls went away. I thoroughly enjoy working in commercial lending at the bank and I love working with the people on my team. The relationships I have developed with my colleagues are a blessing. I am far happier in this environment than I could possibly dream of being at a law firm. This job has opened up possibilities that I did not think would be reality and I hope I can spend my entire working career there.

WHO IS THE BETTER PARENT?

Samantha was with Kendyl in the hospital for the bulk of her stays while I was home with Alyx. We would switch places some weekends so Samantha could come home for a break. This is why we often joked that Alyx was my daughter, Kendyl was hers, and perhaps we would know who the better parent is by seeing how each girl turned out.

All joking aside, I am very happy with how Samantha and I have worked together to raise our girls. Parenting is not an easy task, and it is important for both parents to work together. We have also received a tremendous amount of help from family and friends through this journey and words cannot express how grateful I am for each one of them.

I am also blessed to be married to a woman who is out of my league and that somehow, she is happy with that. I could not ask for anything more. Samantha is a wonderful mother, and I hope that my girls will grow up to be just like her. She is the greatest thing that has ever happened to me and makes up for all of my inadequacies. The better parent between us is not even worth debating.

It was a long journey but just as I said to Samantha on December 11, 2015, I knew everything would be OK. However, it may have been a little different than I thought that day.

LIVEREAL

Yes, Kendyl has had a liver transplant. She received a second chance at life. Yes, she is a special girl and a walking miracle. However, I believe that everyone can have a second chance at life and experience miracles.

I've learned a lot throughout this journey. The phrase "Live Real" has always stuck in my head as it includes the words live, liver, and real. I've learned throughout the years how important it is to live "real" to who you are, what you stand for, and who you want to be. You are created in the image of God and have infinite potential. I hope that by reading Kendyl's story you find the strength and inspiration to believe that.

Are you living up to who you want to be?
If not, start today and LiveReal!

ACKNOWLEDGMENTS

I want to thank Kendyl's amazing liver team at Primary Children's Hospital. I truly believe she has the best doctor and surgeon ever and I won't ever be able to express how much I appreciate this team and what they have done for her and our family. Being close to the liver team throughout the years, I can truly say I love them all (even some who have moved on to different endeavors). Throughout the journey I always felt they truly cared, and I knew my daughter's care was in the best hands. As a parent, this meant the world.

I want to say a big thank you to all our friends, especially those in Spokane who helped tremendously when Kendyl was first diagnosed, and we were living away from family. Thank you for being there for us and for taking good care of Alyx. I don't know what we would have done without you.

I will forever be grateful for our amazing family. While Kendyl was in the hospital over the years, we had lots of family members visiting her and spending time with us. It was amazing to see the team that she had cheering for her and still has today. I hope that someday, as she gets older, I can describe how loved she is and how much support she had through her journey.

Thank you grandma Linda Miller for helping me with editing and being the first to read my work and encouraging me through the process.

My amazing mom, Lisa Jones, thank you for not only being there for me through this journey but also for all your editing help. You took my words and made them better in every way. Not only did you live most of the journey with us, but you also helped to share it in writing.

To my incredible mentor, Danielle Amos, thank you for being an amazing teacher and for your transformational work on my mindset that has changed my life. Thank you for believing in me and encouraging me. Without you, I know this book would not be here. I will be forever grateful for you.

Thank you Eric D. Groleau for your help in making this dream of writing a book about Kendyl's story a reality and for creating what I had pictured in my mind.

Most of all, I want to thank my supportive husband, Zach. I am so proud of you. I don't understand how you managed to take care of us while finishing school. I was and I am still amazed at how you were able to juggle your studies and starting your career when our lives were in complete chaos. I'm still not quite sure how we made it through this journey, but I wouldn't have wanted to go through it with anyone else. I know that I never would have made it through all those hard years without your constant support and love. This experience proves that we can get through anything. Thank you for loving me and the girls. You are the cutest girl dad in the world. I appreciate you supporting and encouraging this book idea and having full confidence in me. I love you babe!

RESOURCES

Become an Organ Donor:

If you have not registered to be an organ donor yet, please consider doing it today. An organ donor can provide life-saving organs to as many as eight people.

Department of Health & Human Services Health Resources & Services Administration (USA)
https://www.organdonor.gov/sign-up

Canadian Organ & Tissue Donors Association (Canada)
https://acdo.ca/index.php/en

TSA Cares:

TSA Cares helps travelers with disabilities, medical conditions and other special circumstances requiring additional assistance during the security screening process. I highly recommend that you contact them at least two weeks before flying with medications or equipment. It makes the process much smoother.

https://www.tsa.gov/travel/passenger-support

Give Kids The World:

Give Kids The World Village is an 89 acre, non-profit resort in Central Florida that provides weeklong, cost-free vacations to children with life-threatening illnesses and their families.

https://www.gktw.org

SALES OF THIS BOOK
WILL HELP SUPPORT

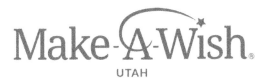

UTAH

Every 20 minutes, a child is diagnosed with a critical illness. Tens of thousands of volunteers, donors and supporters advance the Make-A-Wish® vision to grant the wish of every child diagnosed with a critical illness.

In the U.S. and its territories, a wish is granted every 34 minutes.

A wish can be that spark that helps these children believe that anything is possible and gives them the strength to fight harder against their illnesses. This one belief guides us and inspires us to grant wishes that change the lives of the kids we serve.

https://wish.org

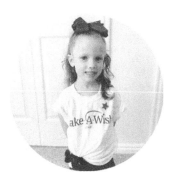

ABOUT THE AUTHOR

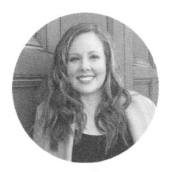

SAMANTHA MELANEY is passionate about living a life of purpose and encouraging others to do the same through physical, mental, and emotional growth. As an author, speaker, and mentor, she uses the lessons learned from her family's journey to inspire people to keep their faith during hard times. She also raises awareness for organ donation by sharing her daughter's story of receiving a lifesaving pediatric liver transplant. Samantha lives with her husband and two beautiful girls in Utah, USA.

.

For more information or to contact Samantha, please visit her website:

SamanthaMelaney.com

ADDITIONAL MATERIALS & RESOURCES

Access your Additional Materials & Resources
referenced throughout this book at
SamanthaMelaney.com/bookbonus

Made in United States
North Haven, CT
16 July 2023

39149697R00137